NATUROPATHY AND YOGA

NATUROPATHY AND YOGA

Parvesh Handa

KALPAZ

Published by

Kalpaz Publications
C-30, Satyawati Nagar,
Delhi – 110052
Ph.: 011-47034999, 9811692060
www.kalpazpublications.com
E-mail: kalpaz@hotmail.com

Distribution Network
gyanbooks.com
India, USA, Canada, UK, Australia, France

ISBN: 978-81-7835-476-7 (HB)

Reprint in India, 2024
First Published, 2006

Printed at: Gyan Press, Delhi.

Naturopathy and Yoga
Author: Parvesh Handa

Contents

Preface

Nature care and Yoga aim at both cure and prevention. Nature care teaches that all treatments work best when the body systems are clean. The principal aspects of Nature Care and Yoga treatments are diet and meditation to eliminate or neutralize toxins. Modern medicines consist mostly antibiotics and chemotherapeutic drugs, which are applied to kill bacteria responsible for production of disease. But these drugs also kill bacterial flora, which is helpful for the maintenance of health and longevity. Yoga and Naturopathy play an important role for an alternative and effective system of medicine, which help to preserve and promote health along with to cure diseases.

Under these treatments, inner and outer beauty are intimately related. The more we nurture ourselves the more radiant and attractive we become outwardly and expressively-irrespective of our body shape and proportions. Thus a well balanced diet, sufficient Yoga exercise, fresh air, plenty of sunlight, pure drinking water, adequate rest and art of living can ensure proper health and prevent disease.

In this book, I have tried to explain Yoga Therapy or treatments for the cure of physical and mental problems. Regularity and punctuality in practicing yogic exercise is the thumb rule. I have also explained Nature Cure basically as a holistic approach, which helps to take proper account of all aspect of health and way of life—that consider nothing in isolation but are connected together. Life is beautiful; let us make it more beautiful by being a Superb Human because a thing of beauty is joy forever.

Parvesh Handa

1

Basics of Naturopathy, Meditation, Pranayama and Yoga

Philosophy of Nature Cure: Naturopathy believes that all diseases are caused due to accumulation of toxins or morbid matter in the body, because of indulgence or ignorance in eating and living habits. These toxins are either exogenous or endogenous. Exogenous toxins are formed in the gut. Animal foods are more toxic than vegetarian food. Endogenous toxins are produced in the body metabolism.

Asthma: Naturopathy Approach: Asthma is characterized by recurrent attacks of dyspnoea with difficult and prolongation of expiratory accompanied by wheezing. The treatment for asthma is given on an intensified method. There are three stages for the treatment i.e. *eliminative, soothing and constructive*. Eliminative stage is directed towards helping the excretory organs, in the elimination of morbid matter from the body. The diet consists mainly of water or diluted fruit juices. Fasting is the health promoting treatment, which stimulates body's inherent power, to fight and promote health. Eliminative treatment include enema, fomentation, chest pack, hot arm bath, plantain leaf pack, asthma bath and back massage. Enema helps in the elimination of morbid matter from the body. Soothing Stage rejuvenate the system by activating the organs. Relaxing moderate exercises, vegetarian diet including fruits and raw vegetables are prescribed during this stage. In Constructive Stage the tissues are rejuvenated, the patient is prescribed high caloric value diet like vegetable soups, sprouted seeds and boiled vegetables. The average intake of food will be 1500 to 2000 calories per day. Constructive treatments include massage, hot and cold hip bath, abdominal and chest pack, steam bath, sun bath and many of the hot water treatments.

Treatments of Yogic Therapy: In addition to nature cure treatment, the asthma patients are exposed to yoga therapy. It can be divided into four inter-related activities such as the Yogic Kriyas, Yogasanas, Pranayama and Laghu Shankap Prakshalana. The yogic kriyas constitute eliminative techniques like Jalaneti, Sutraneti, Kunja and Vastradhouti. The first and second are used for cleansing the nostril and help to clear the blocked nasal passage and eustachin tubes. The regular massage activates the nasal mucosa and makes the mucus membranes of the nose. Kunjal and Vastradhouti are basically stomach washes to get rid of impurities from stomach and clean the chest. The Kunjal (vomiting) relaxes the bronchial wall. Vastradhouti absorbs undesirable bile fluid and gives good massage to the trachea and the stomach. The respiratory troubles are overcome by constant practice of the yogic kriyas. All kriyas will stimulate lungs and bronchia Perform these kriyas in the early morning everyday. These techniques can be learnt in 3 or 4 days.

Yogasanas: Exercise the body muscles, and increase internal organs body strength and provide relaxation to the spine. It stimulates the flow of blood to all parts of the body. This also helps in the elimination of accumulated toxins and waste-product clogged the vital capillaries and the lymphatic and nervous channels. These asanas strengthen the spinal chord and allow the flow of energy into the body. The main asanas prescribed for asthmatic patients are: *Sarvang Asana, Paschimottana Asana, Janusir Asana, Bhujang Asana, Gomukh Asana, Ardhmatsyendra Asana, Padma*

Asana, Baddha Padm Asana, Shalabh Asana, Dhanur Asana, Ustra Asana, Vajra Asana. These asanas are helpful in reshaping the chest and improve body posture. They strengthen the spinal chord and allow the flow of energy into the body. Pranayama is most important for Asthama patients. Pranayama is excellent in lungs diseases. By adding meditation to it, Pranayama can be used for the control of mind. Increases self-confidence. *Anuloma Viloma, Bhastrika, Kapalabhati, Ujjayi and Suryabhedana* are the useful types of paranayama. In Anuloma Viloma normal breathing starts with left nostril and ends with the right. It should be practice every morning and evening. In Bhastrika the respiration is carried out inhaling and exhaling 20 strokes. It has to be carried out 5 times each in the morning and 5 times in the evening. Suryabhedana is practiced using the right nostril only for inhaling and exhaling and should be done just before the attack of asthama. This provides relaxation and produces a soothing effect.

Laghu Shanka Prakshalan: The patient should not take any food before practising this yogic kriya. He/She should be given two glasses of tepid saline water. The patient gets clear bowel movement along with creation of large quantity of urine.

Pranayama: The sanskrit word Prana means 'Vital Force' or 'Cosmic Energy'—which signifies 'life' or 'breath'. Ayama means control of the 'prana'. Thus pranayama means the control of concentration and regular breathing which is essential to life: the absorption of air by inhalation of oxygen and its expulsion by exhaling of carbonic gas. The yogic breathing consists of three parts: the abdomen, thorax (middle part of the chest) and clavicle (upper part of the chest or collar bone). Always inhale and exhale through the nose. The nose is to breathe, the mouth is to eat and to speak.

Pranayama means life, and vice-versa. A new born baby starts breathing just after birth when the lungs are filled with air. Before birth, in the womb of mother the baby does not breathe, but respiration still exists and oxygen is supplied to each cell of the growing body inside the womb. To practice Pranayama, the following rules should be kept in mind:

1. Start Pranayama at the age of eight to ten years.
2. Pranayama is equally useful for both sexes male and females.
3. Practise pranayama in a peaceful, calm, noiseless and airy environments.
4. Wear clothes which are sufficient to protect the body. Avoid wearing tight clothes.
5. Practice pranayama empty stomach, two hours after breakfast and four hours after a meal and an hour after a cup of tea.
6. Start practicing pranayama for a short period and gradually increase the duration.
7. Pranayama practitioner should be a vegetarian as far as possible.

Complete Yogic Breathing: These are of two types:

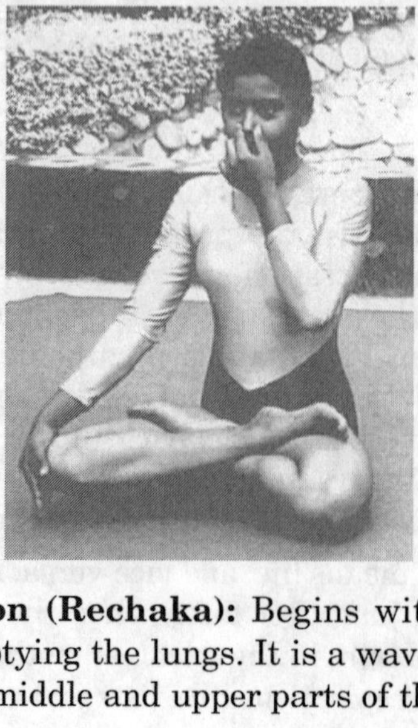

Exhalation (Rechaka): Begins with the abdomen completely emptying the lungs. It is a wave like movement by abdominal, middle and upper parts of the chest.

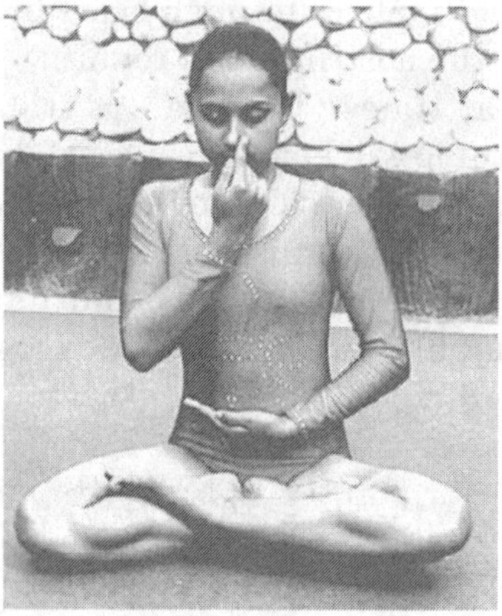

Inhalation (Puraka): After exhalation, begin to inhale and fill the lungs the whole process of inhaling and exhaling should be done as one smooth, continuous movement like a wave.

Benefits: It is important for good health. Should be regarded as a gift from the nature.

- Brings respiratory organs into play and guards against pulmonary infections.
- Prevents asthma and heart trouble.
- Nourishes vital organs, endocrine glands, nervous centres and body tissues.
- Maintains blood pressure in the arteries.
- Calms nervous system.
- Provided mental and physical peace.

Rhythmic Breathing: It has two variations. First: inhalation and exhalation take equal time. Secondly, inhalation and exhalation takes the same amount of time but there is pause between the two equal to half the time each. To perform rhythmic breathing, sit cross-legged holding the chest, neck and head in a straight, vertical line with hands on knees. Inhale counting 6 heart beats, then slowly exhale through the nostrils again counting to 6. Repeat the exercise several times. The therapeutic advantages of Rhythmic breathing will help to revive exhausted body, calm tired nerves, have better sleep, enhances facial beauty (the skin starts glowing and wrinkles softens), relieve the ageing of muscles, bring health to body and mind, help to re-establish the equilibrium of the nervous and neuro-vegetal refreshed the brain.

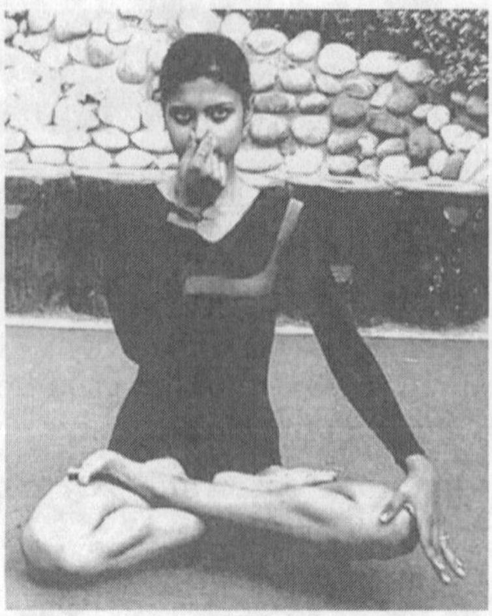

Kumbhaka (Retention of the Breath): Inhale breathing sitting cross legged in Padmasana (Lotus Posture). Hold breath from 6 to 32 seconds. Then exhale following the same rhythm as in case of inhaling. In case of feeling of suffocation or suffering from illness or heart trouble do not perform this exercise. This breathing exercise is very effective for healthy respiratory system, re-establish the equilibrium of position and increase will power, avoid problems of lungs, liver, gallbladder, stomach and heart.

Nadi Shodhana (Alternate Breathing): This practice includes inhaling by the right nostril which produces heat in the body and inhaling by the left nostril which produces cold in the body. To begin with repeat this yogic pranayama not more than three times. Those suffering from cardiac complaints, high blood pressure, weak lungs should avoid practice without consulting a yogic teacher. In this posture sit in Padmasana. Begin exhaling, keeping the index finger or right hand in the centre of forehead between the eyebrows, close the right nostril with the thumb and inhale through the left nostril counting four heart-beats. Hold to a count of 16, then open the right nostril closing the left with middle finger, exhaling through the right nostril. Repeat the exercise on the other side. Nadi-Shodhana Pranayama has therapeutic advantages e.g. establishes the equilibrium to the body, calms and purifies the nerves, cures headache, stabilizes the mind and increases mental power.

Ujjayi (Energy Renewing Pranayama): The exhalation in the pranayana breathing exercise is twice as long as inhalation and holding of the breath. If inhalation is carried for 4 seconds, retention and exhalation should be done for 8 seconds each. The exercise may be performed in sitting or standing position. Once the breath contained in the lungs has been completely exhaled, the air is inhaled through both nostrils. Repeat three times in the beginning and gradually increase the number.

The following Asanas are beneficial in Pranayama:

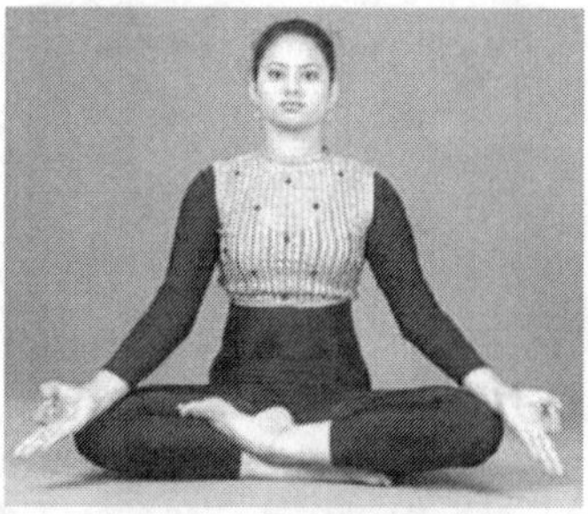

Padma Asana (Lotus Posture): Keep the right foot on the left thigh and left foot on the right thigh. Keep hands on the heels, the back (spinal column) and neck erect.

Padmasana is a widely described as a meditative posture. Therapeutic advantage of this position include developing physical and mental stability, calms the nerves, relieves stiffness of knees and joints, supplies blood to abdominal region and the entire body is kept in complete equilibrium.

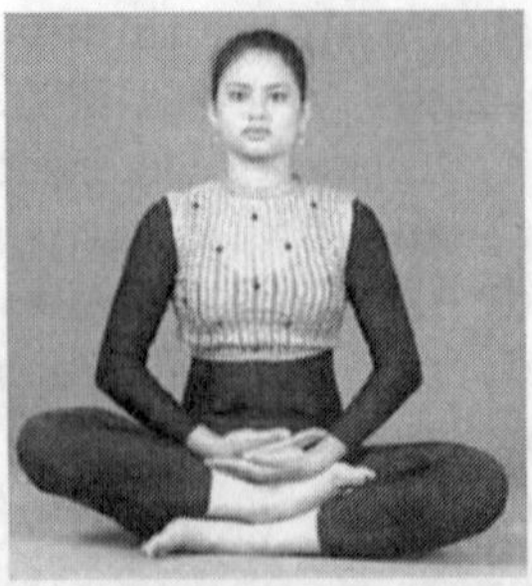

Sidda Asana (Posture of the Adept): In this exercise sit with the left heel set against the perineum and the right heel on the left one. This posture supplies blood to pelvic region and the benefits are similar to padmasana. Take care not to hurt genitals and keep spinal column vertical.

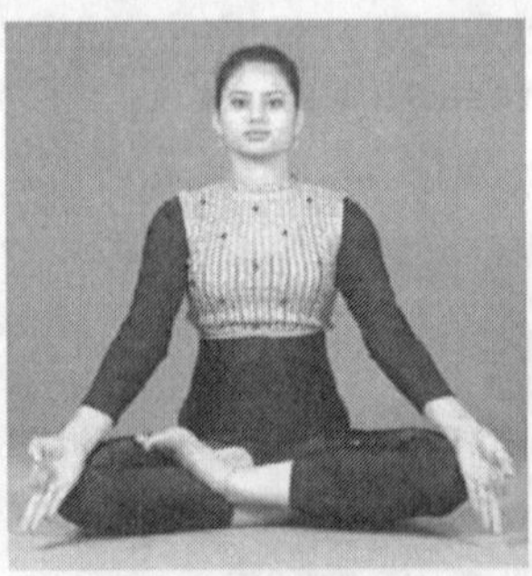

Sukh Asana (Comfortable Posture): This posture is similar to padmasana and therapeutic advantages of both are also identical. Sit at ease with straight back, keeping one foot under the opposite thigh and the other under the opposite leg.

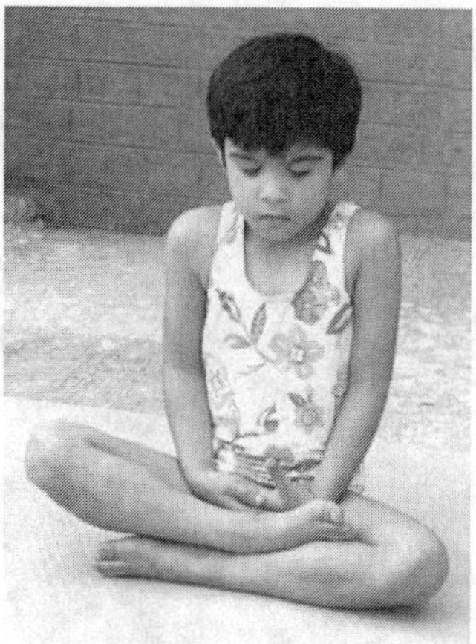

Svastika Asana (The Auspicious Posture): Sit with right heel placed against the left hip and left foot against the right calf. The therapeutic advantages of this posture are identical to those Padmasana.

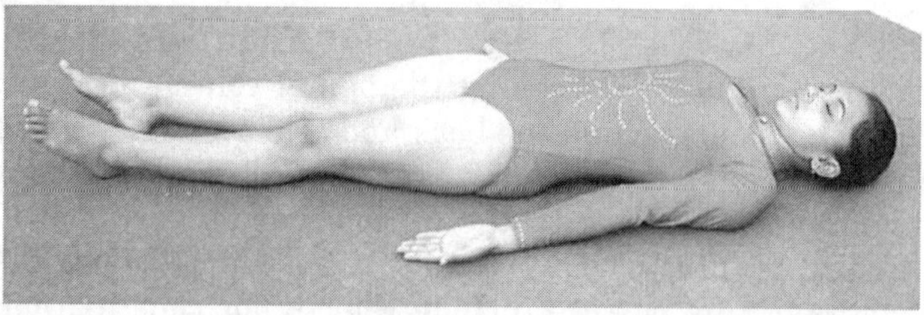

Savasana (Complete Relaxation Posture): In sanskrit sava means 'Corpse' in which one lies on the back like a corpse with relaxed mind and body. In this posture keep arms at the sides, legs stretched out slightly apart, eyes closed, breath rhythmical slowly and deeply. Keep the brain completely empty. The benefits include calm heart and nervous system. It cures high blood pressure, insomnia, nervous disorders, depression, eliminate the toxins accumulating in the blood, recharge energy and regenerate body cells.

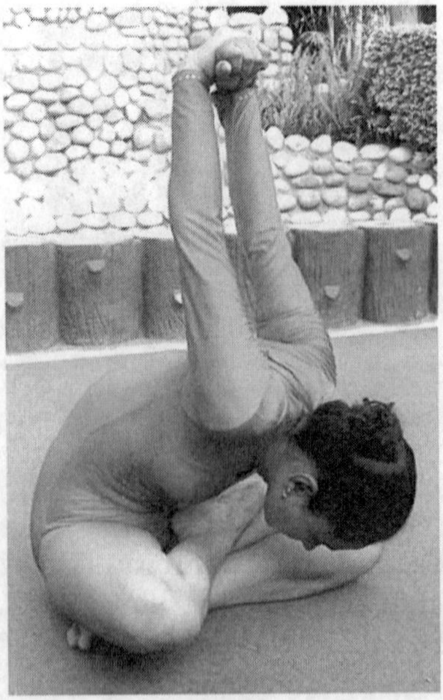

Yog Mudra (The Symbol of Yoga): Sit in the Padmasana position keeping the spinal column upright. Place the hands behind the back and grab the wrist of one hand with the other hand. Lean forward gently without straining one hand with the other. Lear forward gently without straining or jerking the spinal column. Among the benefits of this posture include remedy for constipation, toning up the abdominal muscles/organs, exercise the lungs, help flow of blood from the lower region to upwards, has a curative effect for the asthmatics, correct disorders of the spine, strengthen the digestive system and enhance sexual potentiality.

Uddiyana Bandha (Raising of Diaphragm): In Sanskrit, uddiyana means 'to raise' and Bandha means 'contraction'. This posture is similar to Nauli. Expand chest without allowing the air to enter the lungs after exhaling deeply. This will pull the diaphragm upward in the thoracic cavity, pulling back abdominal wall. In this posture stand with legs 12 to 18 inches apart, knees slightly bent and pressing hands on the thigh and try to bring the abdominal wall far back towards. Doing this posture is excellent to prevent gastric complaints, dyspepsia, liver problem, to remove toxins from digestive tract, to prevent fat deposits around the waist and abdomen. Avoid this yogic exercise, if you suffer from abdominal complaint, prolapses of stomach, uterus or intestines.

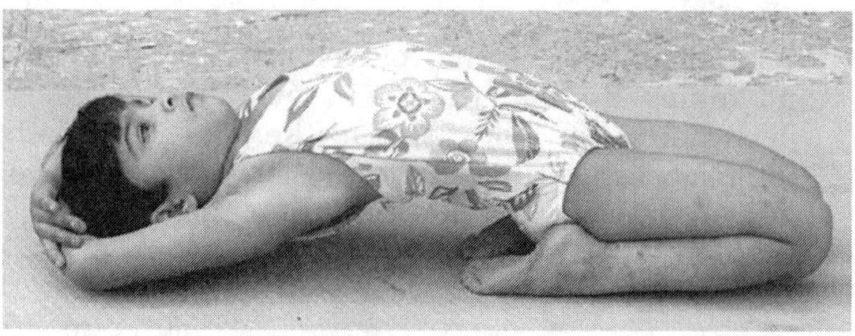

Supta Vajar Asana (The Supine Pelvic Posture): Vajra means lighting. A sitting posture in which the thighs are arranged in the form of a vajra. Sit between the heels not on them as Muslim's sit for their Namaz prayers. Lean backward slowly until back of the head rest on the ground, placing hands under the mape of neck. Relax for 6-8 seconds, then return to Vajra asana. Repeat the exercise 3-4 times. This asana strengthens male and female sex organs, cures indigestion, wind trouble, piles and constipation.

Warming up Exercises: Warming up exercises are essential before starting yoga practice for a shapely figure and to obtain perfect results. Brisk walk in the fresh morning air is very beneficial. Brisk walk gives exercise to entire body, especially useful for hips and thighs. Outdoor games and swimming too are useful for tautness of muscles. Warming up exercises before practicing yoga prevent accumulation of fat. Following are some useful tips:

- Always cool down after a yoga session with slow, gentle

stretches. When you begin to feel more poised, loose limbed, coordinated, stretched and toned, feel like as if you are gliding rather walking. These come from the muscles of the body loosening, growing more elastic and strong, Warming up exercises help disappearance of aches and discomforts in bones and burden off your joints.

- If you are extremely overweight, about 20 kg or above your standard weight or have strain, pain and inflammation in joints—do not run, walk or do lunges. These weight bearing exercises strain your joints even more. Instead, go for about 30 minutes stationary cycling (instanding)—it does not put pressure on your knees and ankles. It stimulates the synovia fluid in the body which helps self lubrication in the joints. In another stationary self-cycling exercise when lie down on your back, move your legs like cycling motion for 10 to 15 minutes.
- Exercise at least two hours after a meal. Two hour gap helps the body to digest food properly. This will help, you do not get muscle cramps or gas from half digested food.
- Pre-exercise meal should be light. Soup and salad for lunch makes an ideal and delightful exercise. If you feel over- stimulated after exercising and disturb your sleep at night, reduce your exercising time and movements. These are symbols of overdoing exercise. A good deep exercise where you wake up refreshed is a sign of healthy exercising schedule according to comfortable requirement.
- Wear cotton socks while walking or running, which absorb perspiration. Avoid wearing socks and thick heeled shoes when doing yoga exercises. Also wear loose cotton clothes to allow your body to breathe.
- Cool down after exercising a session with slow and gentle stretches. Stopping exercise abruptly makes blood circulation faulty, that start rapid circulation of blood pumping in reverse direction and give puffy feelings in the lower region of the body.

- Consult a doctor before embarking on an yogic exercise programme, especially when you are over 40 years of age, if you have a personal or family history of high blood pressure or heart problem.
- Too much and too fast yogic practice does not provide instant results—these simply lead to injuries, aches and pains. Slow start exercise programme is harmful as body muscles need to be conditioned gradually. Increase practice of yogic exercise gradually for a pleasure instead of discomfort. Exercise to your favourite music or in a group. These ease stress.

Therapeutic Yoga-Harmony of Body and Mind: Yoga is a system of self treatment of diseases, disorders and ailments as a result of faulty ways of living, bad habits, lack of proper knowledge, imporper food and malfunctioning of the body system. 'Ayurved'—'Ayu' and 'Veda' means the science of life, and has eight branches i.e. Kayachikitsa (general medicine), Shalya (Surgery), Shalakya (treatment of head, eye, neck and throat), Graha Chikitsa (pyschotherapy), Damstra chikitsa (toxicology), Bala Roga Chikitsa (Paediatrics), Jara Chikitsa (Rejuvenation), Vrishya Chikitsa (Aphrodisiacs). The universe is composed of five basic elements viz., Prithvi, Ap, Tejas, Vayu and Akasha. Water, Fire and Air are the essential substances for the human body. Ayurveda believes in the theory of tridoshas by Vata, Pitta and Kapha. Vata is a powerful force in the body produced by the combination of Vayu and Akasha, Kapha is produced due to the predominance of Earth and Water, Pitta is produced due to predominance of Tejas.

The Eight-Fold Path-Ashtanga Yoga: Ashta means eight and anga means limbs. The eight limbs of Yoga are:

- **Yama:** Refers to Ahimsa (Non-violence), Satya (Truth), Asteya (Non-stealing), Brahmacharya (Self-control) and Aparigraha (Unselfishness).
- **Niayma:** Which refers to Saucha (Cleanliness), Santosha (Contentment), Tapas (Effort), Svadhyaya

(Self Study) and Ishvara Pranidhana (Faith in God).

- **Asana:** Means posture.
- **Pranayama:** Means control of the senses e.g. taste, touch, smell, sight and hearing.
- **Dharana:** Means concentration.
- **Dhyana:** Means meditation.
- **Samadhi:** Means samadhi that unites with God.

Adopting these means eight-fold paths control over health of body and control over mind. For children, only yama, niyama and asana are important. The girls during their menstrual period should never do upside down poses such as *Shirsha Asana. Sarvanga Asana, Hala Asana, Karnapida Asana, Adho Mukha Vriksha Asana, etc.* However consult your teacher for correct posture. Children below 8 years of age will not be able to perform asanas such as *Shirsha Asana, Sarvanga Asana, Hala Asana and Karna pida Asana* due to their under developed body. Don't force yourself to breathe deeply or to hold your breath while doing the asanas. Breathe normally, always through the nose. Always be alert, attentive and watchful when you practice. Concentrate on your pose.

2

Drugless Therapies

Depression is the most prevalent of all the emotional disorders. This may vary from feelings of slight sadness to utter misery and brings together a variety of physical and psychological symptoms. Depression is the most unpleasant experience a person can endure. The growing complexities of modern life and the resulting crisis, mental stress and strain in day-to-day living usually lead to this disorder. Suicide is the major risk in extreme cases of depression. The most striking symptoms of depression are feelings of acute sense, sadness, loss of energy, constipation, loss of appetite giddiness, tiredness, sleep disturbance, insomnia, nightmares, repeated waking from midnight onwards, itching, nausea, agitation, irritability, impotence and frigidity, aches and pains in the body, low body temperature, low blood pressure, rapid loss of weight, hot flushes and sensation of shivering and loss of interest. The following are the main causes of mental depression:

1. Depleted functioning of the adrenal glands.
2. Irregular diet habits cause digestive problems and lead to the assimilation of fats. Gases produced due to indigestion cause compression over the region of the heart and lungs.
3. The excessive and indiscriminate use of drugs leads to faulty assimilation of vitamins and minerals and causes depression.

4. An excessive intake of fats may also lead to depression.

The modern medical system treats depression with anti-depression drugs which provide temporary relief and leave a harmful side -effect. The harmful side-effects which include liver damage, hypersensitivity, insomnia, hallucinations, low blood pressure, headaches and dizziness, blurred vision, difficulty in inhaling and urine retention. Naturopathy treatment of depression consists of regulating the diet, yogic exercise, scientific relaxation and meditation. The diet of persons suffering from depression should completely exclude tea, coffee, alcohol, chocolate and cola, all white flour products, sugar, food colourings, white rice and strong condiments. The diet should be restricted to three meals. Exercise also plays an important role in the treatment of depression. It not only keeps the body physically and mentally fit but also provides recreation and mental relaxation. It is nature's best tranquillizer. Exercise produces chemical and psychological changes that improve mental health. It changes the levels of hormones in blood and may elevate mood affecting brain chemicals. Some of the yogic asanas such as *Bhujangasana (Cobra Pose), Halasana (Plough Pose), Dhanurasana (Bow Pose), Sarvangasana (Shoulder-Stand Pose), Virbhadra Asana, and Pranayamas* are highly beneficial in the treatment of depression.

Relaxation: The patient needs control over his nervous system and channelise his mental emotional activities into restful harmonious vibrations, which can be achieved by sufficient rest and sleep. Learn the art of scientific relaxation and meditation, which will go a long way in curing depression. Relaxation enables the muscles to work efficiently and eliminates fatigue by promoting blood circulation in the body. The best method of relaxation is to practice **Savasana** or the 'dead pose'. Meditation will help create an amount of balance in the nervous system, enable the glands to return to a correct state of hormonal balance and thereby overcome depression.

A Neutral Immersion Bath: It is also known as "Full Bath" is also helpful in the treatment of depression. This bath is administered in a bath tub which should be properly fitted with hot and cold water connection. The patient should lie in the tub filling it with water at a particular temperature. The head should be kept cold with a cold compress.

A Cold Immersion Bath: May be taken in a tub for 4 to 20 minutes at a temperature ranging from 10.00 to 23.80° C. Cold water should be poured on the patient's head, chest and the neck before entering the bath. After the bath, the body should be dried and wrapped up in a blanket. The bath also helps to bring down fever, improves the skin, acute peritonitis, gastritis, enteritis and inflammatory conditions of uterus and ovaries.

Hot Immersion Bath: Should be taken from 5 to 15 minutes at a temperature from 36 to 40°C. The temperature can be gradually raised to the required level by adding hot water. Before entering bath the patient should drink cold water and also wet his head, neck and shoulders with cold water. This bath gives relief to congestion of the lungs and activates the blood vessels of the skin muscles. After the bath, apply oil. The hot bath treats obesity, chronic rheumatism and the pain due to stones in the gall bladder and the kidney.

Cold Compress: The cloth should be dipped in cold water or ice water. The compress is generally applied to the head, neck, chest, abdomen and back. The cold compress is effective means of controlling inflammatory conditions of lever, spleen, stomach, kidneys, intestines, lungs, brain, pelvic organs, fever and heart disease.

Heating Compress: Consists of three to four folds of linen cloth wrung out in cold water, is then covered with blanket to prevent circulation of air and accumulation of body heat, can be applied to the root, chest and abdomen.

Sleep: It is nature greatest blessing of life which repairs the wear and tear of the body and mind. Nothing is so restorative to the nerves as sound and uninterrupted sleep. The amount of sleep needed for an individuals well being, is determined by what he needs. On the whole most of the women sleep from 45 minutes to 60 minutes more than men. The amount of sleep required varies at different ages as below:

New Born: 18 to 20 hours.

Growing Children: 10 to 12 hours

Adults: 7 to 9 hours

Aged Persons: 5 to 7 hours

For proper sleep, however one should not sleep on one's back but on the side with one or both legs brought well up and the head and the shoulders slightly forward. The sleeping place should be well ventilated, with balanced temperature and free from noises. The bed should be neither too hard or too soft, but comfortable. The pillow should not be too hard or too high.

Insomnia: Insomnia or sleeplessness has alarming effect among the upper classes in the urban. Insomnia deprives the person of mental rest. Sleep give relief from tension, rests the brain and body and the amount of sleep varies from individual to individual. Normally, seven to eight hours of sleep every night is adequate.

The most common cause of sleeplessness are mental tension, anxiety, worries, overwork, overexcitement, dull brain, suppressed feelings of resentment, anger and bitterness, constipation, dyspepsia, over-eating, excessive intake of tea or coffee, smoking and going to bed hungry increase the problem as these irritate the nervous system, especially the nerves of the digestive system. Sleeping pills are not recommended for sleeplessness. The side effects of sleeping pills include indigestion, skin rashes, lowered resistance to infection, circulatory and respiratory problems and mental confusion.

Ten Step to Relieve Insomnia

1. Have a regular sleeping schedule; going to bed at a fixed time at night and getting up at a fixed time morning. Early to bed and early to rise is a good practice.
2. Deficiencies of key nutrients such as B-complex vitamins and vitamin C and D, calcium, magnesium, potassium and zinc cause Insomnia.
3. A balanced diet and the eating pattern will go a long way in the treatment of insomnia. Exclude white flour products, sugar and its products, tea, coffee, chocolate, cola drinks, alcohol, fatty foods, fried foods, foods containing additives, excessive use of salt and strong condiments.
4. It is better to divert the mind with soft music or light reading while going to bed.
5. Use light bed clothes and relax.
6. Do not lie on your back, but on your side with one or both knees brought well up and the head and shoulders slightly forward. The position of the arms and legs should be changed frequently.
7. Controlled breathing also help in inducing sleep. Lie on your side and take three deep breaths, expanding the abdomen completely. Then hold your breath as long as you can. Take three more breaths and repeat the breath-holding. While you hold breath, carbon dioxide accumulates in the body and induces natural sleep.
8. Have regular exercise during the day and mild exercise at bedtimes, this will help to enhances the quantity and the quality of sleep. Exercise stimulates, eliminates lactic acid from the body relieves stress and muscular tension, produces hormonal changes beneficial to the body and sleep pattern. Walking, jogging, skipping, cycling and swimming are ideal exercise.
9. Yoga helps a majority of cases of insomnia and tones up

the glandular, respiratory and nervous system. The yogasanas effective for insomnia include Sarvangasana, Halasana and Shavasana.

10. Application of hot spinal packs, hot fomentation to the spine, hot footbath, immersion bath before retiring at night are all beneficial to overcome insomnia.

Along with the various measures for the treatment of insomnia, all efforts should be made to eliminate as many stress factors as possible. The measures taken in this regard include regular practice of any relaxation method or meditation technique, cultivating the art of doing things slowly, particularly activities like eating, walking and talking.

Role of Chromotherapy: The sun looks white, but it has the seven colours: violet, indigo, blue, green, yellow, orange and red—out of which violet, indigo and blue are creating cool effect on the body and are also antiseptic. The three colours yellow, orange and red create heath. The remaining green colour is neutral. Chromotherapy is very effective for chronic and dreaded diseases. The effect of different colours on various disease is listed below:

Violet: Bones, tumour, baldness, cataract blindness.

Indigo: Eye-nose-throat problems, facial paralysis, disease of lungs, asthma, tuberculosis, indigestion, problems of nerves system, convulsion, madness.

Blue: Whooping cough, throat problem, cholera, typhoid, small-pox, measles, mouth ulcer, swelling in brain, problems of nerves, insomnia, mental depression, problems of semen discharge, nose bleeding, premature ejaculation and used as antiseptic.

Green: Heart troubles lever problems, high blood pressure, syphilis (venereal disease), inflammation in eyes.

Yellow: Disorders of digestion, spleen and liver problems, diabetes and leprosy.

Orange: Asthma, bronchitis, swelling in trachea, gout, kidney swelling, mental nervousness, epilepsy.

Red: Anaemia, disability, sluggishness, paralysis, white spots, arthritis, T.B. etc.

Ninety minutes after the sunrise and 60 minutes before the sun set take sunrays. Keep the glass of desired colour in the sunlight in such a way that the rays will fall on the affected parts. While taking sunlight, care should be taken that the patient is not exposed to strong direct wind. If sunlight is not possible, take a 60 to 100 watts coloured bulb. In case such colored bulb is not available, take a plain bulb and wrap colored gelatin paper around it. Keep affected part about 20 inches away and have the light for 5 to 10 minutes twice a day.

To take colours through water, have a glass bottle of the desired colour or wrap gelatin paper of the desired colour on the white glass bottle. Fill it 3/4 th with water and keep it in sunlight for at least 3 hours between 10 a.m and 3 p.m. Takecare, the coloured water is not exposed to any other type of colours. This colour-medicated water can be given to the patient at an interval of 15 minutes to two hours depending upon the intensity of the disease.

The Rejunvenation Therapies: Siddha Vaidya and Ayurveda use special herbalized oils and herbs that trigger changes in mind and organs of the body to bring balance and harmony to the overall system. The herbs called adaptogens not only provide nutritional support, balance but modify systems of the body. These adaptogens react in the body that is appropriate to achieve a state of homeostasis or balance. They affect the autonomic nervous system, the endocrine system and the blood pressure. Adaptogens are credited with these properties. Help the body adapt to stress, achieve body balance, increase protein biosynthesis, elevate body enzymes synthesis, promote general endocrine synthesis, improve mental power, increase physical ability, fight free radicals, improve eyesight, beneficial to cardiovascular and respiratory system and improve specific resistance to various stressors like heat, cold, wind. The following naturopathic therapies are beneficial:

Shirodhara: Thin thread of warmed oil is poured over the forehead and scalp. Shirodhara calms the mind, pacifies vatha, cleanses, calms and balances the nervous system, relieves stress and improves mental clarify. Shirodhara improves the body's heat and is used before the rejuvenation (Kriya Karma) therapies. Shirodhara is usually repeated three to four times a week for optimal benefit.

Nasaya: It is a procedure aimed at reducing waste products from the head, throat and nose in human body. Nasaya is the introduction of medicated substances into the nose, stimulates secretion, remove impurities of the head and neck. The treatments primary effect is to improve the connection between different organs of perception. Nasaya is used in headaches, sinusitis, nervousness, migraines, vascular headache, stiff neck, running eyes, ear infections, hearing loss, tinnitus (ringing in ears), loss of smell, and much more. This treatment can be used several times a week in conjuction with other therapies like reflexology and head massage.

Rasayanas: Means rejuvenate system and tissue—is a beneficial treatment for the face and scalp to encompass a head to toe beauty along with other treatments such as massage (abhyanga), steam (svedana), use of the herbs, pastes and masques (snehana), foot reflexology, face and scalp treatments aromatherapy, colour therapy, crystals and gems are used in preparation for Pancha Karma (cleasning and strengthening) and Kriya Karma (rejuvenation). These are the therapies and body treatments that leave your skin looking and feeling fresh and healthy. Purva Karma is also used for maintaining health which helps Pancha Karma or Kriya Karma treatments.

Siddha Massage: Promotes relaxation, calming of Vitha, Kapha and Pittha. It balances and increases the circulation to body's largest eliminative organ the skin. It also aids and facilitates the removal of waste products into the central circulation from where it is removed. It increases lymph flow, strengthens the immune system and relieves muscle tension. The mobility of the ligaments, tendons and joints is increased, thereby adding to the flexibility of the body organs besides helping to calm, relax, tone and balance nervous system. It can be used to treat sleeplessness. Siddha massage regulates the other systems and organs such as the digestive and eliminative system known to increase the production of collagen and elastin fibers, aids in the removal and preventing wrinkling, increases suppleness of the skin besides to relieve muscle spasm and pain of chronic/acute origin.

Abyanga: It is recommended for muscle soreness, joint pain and stiffness, nervousness, tension, stress, lack of energy, restlessness, immune dysfunction, fatigue and tiredness, paralysis/paresis of traumatic origin injury, poor digestion, poor elimination, sleeplessness and ungrounded feelings.

Sandalwood Treatments: It is best suited for water retention, is diuretic and diaphoretic, leads to detoxification, stress reduction. Cellulite triggers skin to sweat and release toxins and acts as disinfectant. Sandalwood has been used for centuries in meditation and medicine. It creates spiritual cleansing as well as cleansing the physical body. Sandalwood increases merely a sense of well-being and is used as an aphrodisiac. Sandalwood unlocks trapped fluids and toxins been stored in the tissues and is a disinfectant and astringent.

Panch Karma means '5 action': It is an ancient scientific system for detoxification. It rejuvenates the whole system, bringing youthfulness and strength in the body and calms openness to the mind. Traditionally, it is undertaken as preventive therapy at the change of season, the aim to cleanse the body not only of waste materials in the body but also excessive in subtle energies or tissues, thereby promoting positive health and longevity through the changing climatic conditions.

Shiatsu Therapy: This therapy, also known as acupressure, is used to treat disorders by pressing various pressure points on the skin of body. There are nearly 600 shiatsu points on the human body and we shall discuss few very important to cure disorders. Pressure on such points produces energy that flows in the body. It takes about 45 to 60 minutes to treat whole body. Shiatsu treatments are given on the floor. Lie face down on a towel. Keep both hands moving rhythmically along the meridians from one point to the other pressing on each point from three to seven seconds. When breathing out, run down either side of spine. It takes about 45 to 60 minutes to treat the whole body, which improves the circulation and induce relaxation. The following steps are carried out to practice shiatsu:

1. Press down either side of the spine.
2. Use the heels of hand, then repeat with thumbs.
3. Press down the buttocks and the back of the legs with light pressure over the knees.
4. Squeeze down pressing on the points on the arms and hands, and the front of the legs.
5. Press gently on all points on the abdomen working clockwise in circles.
6. Work from the centre of the chest outwards, pressing in lines between the ribs.

How to Use Massage Oil?: Do not pour the oil directly to the body. Pour about a teaspoon oil into the palm of one hand. Rub hands, then stroke the oil on the body. Massage with essential oils is very useful for the skin, vigour and vitality. Some people with excessive oily skin use talcum powder for a dry massage. Use a light vegetable oil scented with few drops of essential oil.

Table I

Shiatsu Point in Front of Body Relieving Effects On

1. Lungs, Chest and cough: Press grooves between ribs.
2. To ease tension: Press shoulder muscles.
3. Tired arm and hand muscles: Below elbow crease on arms.
4. Body pain and restore energy: Press shin bone under knees.
5. Alleviates menstrual problems and constipation: Press abdomen at the centre.
6. Headaches (pregnant should avoid): Press between thumb and index finger.
7. Stimulates circulation and relaxed tired legs: Press outer of thighs below waistline.
8. Ease menstrual paint and labour problems: Press groove behind shin bone.

Table II

Shiatsu Point in Back of Body Relieving Effects On

1. Headache, backache and fatigue: Press crown of head.
2. Headache, cold, sinus and nosebleed: Press base of the skull.
3. Strengthens heart, lungs, digestion and reproductive organs: Muscles on the spine.
4. Mensuration pain and backache: Centre of the abdomen.
5. Stomach pain and relaxes body: One inch above or below navel.
6. Energising whole body: On the back, at waistline level.
7. Weight reduction, cellulite: On front, 3 inches below navel.

Reflex Point on the Face: They improve the circulation and energy flow in the face and tone the skin.

Hold each point for five seconds applying pressure at:

If Suffering from Headache and Migraines

- Centre of hairline to the crown of head.
- Centre between the eyebrows.
- On top edge of cheekbone just below the eye.
- Below the end of eyebrows.

If Suffering from Overweight

- On the centre of groove between nose and upper lip.

If Suffering from Tired Eyes, Eye Bags and Puffy Eyes

- Inner corner of the eyes.
- Middle of eyebrows.
- Between eye sockets and cheekbones.

If Suffering from Facial Tension, Nasal Congestioned and Toothache

- Small grooves at the side of the nose.

If Suffering from Tired or Sagging Face

- Centre for lower cheekbone.
- Outer corners of the eyes.
- Hollows just below the ears.

For Energising the Whole Body

- Massage at the centre of the palms of hands.
- In the middle of eyebrows.

Aroma Therapy—A Holistic Therapy

It is a powerful healing art that has profound effect on both body and mind. Aromatherapy makes use of the essential oils, which are extracted from the plants. Essential oil can therefore be absorbed either through the sense of smell or if massaged into the body then through the pores of the skin. Essential oils are highly volatile, evaporating readily on exposure to air and when inhaled may enter the body. When diluted and applied externally, essential oil molecules enter the skin. All essential oils appear to be antiseptic and bactericidal to some extent and may also be helpful in treatment of viral infection. These essential oils have the potential to stimulate healthy cell renewal and growth and to regulate and restore balance to mind body systems.

Essential oils are the aromatic or volatile constituents found in plants. Most essential oils are light sensitive, heat sensitive, very fluid, highly concentrated and have a characteristic fragrance. Essential oils are produced in different parts of plants e.g. roots, leaves, flowers, fruits, seeds, peel and bark and usually extracted by Steam Distillation. There are three ways in which essential oil molecules enter the body and have an effect on it by inhalation, transdermal absorption and ingestion. Aromatherapy increases blood supply to the tissues, which aid to beauty.

Effect on the Body and Mind: Essential oils have a therapeutic effect on the body as they are analgesic; anti-fungal; anti-inflammatory; antioxidant; antiseptic; anti-spasmodic; antiviral; catmant; carminative; depurative; digestive; diuretic; expectorant; hepatic; laxative; hypertensive and hypotensive; sedative; stimulant; toning and many more. Essential oils restore balance to the emotions and mind. It soothes nervous tension and settle a worried mind, calms anxiety and apprehension, improves concentration and memory, boosts moral and pacifies anger and frustration, uplifts depression and negativity, enhances love and relationship and strengthens the spirit to help indecision. Essential oils are absorbed by the body through massage or hydrotherapy. They penetrate the skin and the lining of the lungs to be carried around the body in the blood.

Massage, together with aromatherapy provide the following benefits:

1. Induce deep relaxation, relieving both physical and mental fatigue.
2. Improve circulation to the muscles, thus reducing inflammation and pain.
3. Release neck and shoulder tension and backache.
4. Relieve neuralgic, arthritic and rheumatic conditions.
5. Help sprains, fractures, breaks and dislocations heal readily.
6. Promote correct posture and improve mobility.
7. Improve the function of every internal organ.
8. Improve digestion, assimilation and elimination and also relive constipation.
9. Increase the ability of the kidneys to function efficiently.
10. Flushes the lymphatic system by the mechanical elimination of harmful substances including toxins from bacteria and waste matter.
11. Reduce high blood pressure.
12. Help disperse headaches or migraines
13. Compensate for lack of active exercise.
14. Stimulate mind and body without any side effects.
15. Help release suppressed feelings.
16. Stimulate the immune system.

Essential Oil Therapy: Essential oils penetrate deep into the layers of the skin. Due to their nourishing, cleansing and detoxifying qualities these oils tighten the skin, increase blood circulation, calm the nervous system and support the skin's functions. Essential oils should always be diluted into a steam bath, a compress, bath oil, body or skin lotion or massage oil.

Choose Appropriate Essential Oils for Different Skin-Types

Normal Skin: Camomile, geranium, jasmine, neroli, rose, ylang-ylang.

Troubled Skin (Irritated): Cedar wood, eucalyptus, peppermint, rosemary.

Oily Skin: Bergamot, camphor, cedarwood, cypress, geranium, juniper berry, lavender, lemon, rosewood, sandalwood, vetiver.

Dry Skin: Camomile, clary sage, geranium, lavender, jasmine, neroli, orange, patchouli, rose, rosewood, sandalwood, vetiver.

Rough, Broken Skin: Camomile, lavender, rose, sandalwood.

Broken Veins: Camomile, lavender, neroli, rose, rosewood.

Edemas: Camomile, birch, clary sage, fennel, juniperberry, cypress, orange, peppermint, rosemary, neroli.

Acne: Camphor, bergamont, cypress, cedarwood, camomile, eucalyptus, geranium juniper berry, lavender, lemon, peppermint, rosemary, thyme, sandalwood.

Sensitive Skin: Camomile, geranium, jasmine, neroli, rose, rosewood.

Inflamed Skin: Camomile, clary sage, geranium, jasmine, neroli, sandalwood.

Mature and Aging Skin: Blue camomile, clary sage, cypress, frankincense, lavender, fennel, neroli, orange, rose, rosewood, sandalwood, vetiver, ylang-ylang.

Cellulite: Birch, cypress, juniper berry, lemon, orange, rosemary.

Psoriasis: Bergamot, lavender, neroli.

Stretch marks: They are small tears on the skin surface at first as red or purplish marks which eventually fade to a colour lighter than your skin. They are caused by rapid weight-gain. Essential oils can minimize the scarring of the skin. Massage or oil body with essential oils once a day, specially at stomach, breast and thighs. Best oils for this condition are frankincense and tangerine, rose, camomile, neroli, sage and rosewood.

Essential Oils—That Heal Skin

Sweet Basil (Ocimum Basilicum): Slightly liquorice aroma: It stimulates mental concentration, strengthens nervous system, revitalises the skin, useful antiseptic and cures respiratory infection when blended with Bergamot, Clary sage and Geranium.

Bay (Pimenta Racemosa): Powerful sweet scent: It stimulates hair growth, relieves muscle spasm, improves circulation, relieves melancholy and nervous exhaustion when blended with Rosemary, Geranium, Lavender, Ylang Ylang and Citrus oils.

Bay Laurel (Laurus Nobilis): Srong, sweet-spicy scent: It regulates the lymphatic system, stimulates the mind, heals bronchitis, relieves sinus infection and melancholy when blended with Lavender, Clary sage, Cypress and Frankincense.

Bergamot (Citrus Bergamia): Strong, sweet-spicy scent: It balances nervous system, relieves anxiety and stress, lifts melancholy, helps restful sleep, antiviral cures cold sores, cures psoriasis and eczema and relieves post-natal stress when blended with Lavender, Neroli, Jasmine, Coriander, Juniper, Camomile and Lemon.

Black Pepper (Piper Nigrum): Warm, peppery aroma. It has energizing effect, increases circulation, relieves muscle aches and stiffness, fights cold and infections, relieves rheumatism and relieves arthritic pain when blended with Rosemary, Lavender, Frankincense, Sandalwood, Marjoram.

Atlas Cedar (Cedrus Allantica): A woody aroma. It relaxes tense muscles, calms emotions, enhances meditation, eases pain and relieves hair loss when blended with

Bergamot, Cypress, Rosemary, Juniper, Vetiver, Neroli, Clary sage.

Roman Camomile (Anthemis Nobilis): Sweet and fruity aroma. It relieves muscular pain, used as a sedative, relieves nervous tension, helps sleeplessness, used as an anti-inflammatory, relieves aches and pains and cures sunbrun and rashes when blended with Bergamot, Jasmine, Cypress, Neroli, Vetiver, Rosemary, Clary sage.

Citronella (Cymbopogon Nardus): Grassy-woody scent. It relieves arthritis pain, cures digestive troubles and soothes and deodorise foot when blended with Geranium, Lemon, Orange, Bergamot.

Clary Sage (Salvia Sclarea): A spicy, hay-like aroma. It relieves stress and tension, eases pain, provides restful sleep, relieves nervous exhaustion, relaxes body muscles, promotes oestrogen hormones and suitable for menopause when blended with Juniper, Lavender, Bergamot, Cypress, Jasmine, Geranium, Sandalwood.

Coriander (Coriandrum Sativum): Spicy, sweet fragrant aroma. It relieves muscular pain and helps nervous exhaustion when blended with Ginger, Bergamot, Jasmine, Neroli, Sandalwood, Cardamon, Sandalwood and Marjoram.

Cypress (Cupressus Semperviren): Spicy, refreshing aroma. It increases circulation, relieves muscular cramps and painful periods, cures bronchitis and whooping cough, reduced nervous tension, used in footbath and relieves aching legs when blended with Cedarwood, Lavendar, Cardamon, Sandalwood, Bergamot, Orange, Clary sage.

Eucalyptust (Eucalyptus Globolus): Strong camphorous odour. It relieves asthma.

Fennel (Foeniculum Vulgare): An earthy-peppery aroma. It relieves neuro muscular spasms, cures arthritis and relieves bronchitis and cough, relieves stress and tension, cures ingestion and constipation, cellulitis and balances female reproductive system when blended with Lavender, Geranium, Rose, Sandalwood.

Frankincense (Boswellea Species): A spicy, aroma. It elevates mind and spirit, calms nerves of body, enhances meditation, relieves respiratory inspections, psychic cleansing, cures scars and boils, clears lines and wrinkles, anti-inflammatory and relieves mouth ulcers when blended with Sandalwood, Pine, Lavendar, Vetiver, Geranium, Neroli, Orange, Bergamot, Basil.

Geranium (Pelargonium Graveolens): A leafy rose scent. It reduces stress and tension, eases pain, balances hormones, relieves fatigue and exhaustion, tones liver and kidney and lifts melancholy when blended with Lavender, Patchouli, Clave, Neroli, Sandalwood, Jasmine.

Ginger (Zingiber Officinale): A warm, spicy woody odour. It reduces muscular pain, increases circulation, relieves bronchitis, cures whooping cough, nervous exhaustion, heals cold and fever and stimulates appetite when blended with Sandalwood, Vetiver, Patchouli, Frankincense, Cedarwood, Coriander, Rose, Neroli, Orange.

Grape Fruit (Citrus Paradist): Fresh, sweet, citrus scent. It relieves muscular aches, increases circulation, relieves bronchitis and stimulates appetite when blended with Lemon, Palmarosa, Rosemary, Geranium, Lavender, Cypress, Neroli, Bergamot.

Jasmine (Jasminum): A rich, sweet scent. It relieves muscular spasm and painful periods, labour pain and anxiety, exhaustion and maintain healthy skin when blended with Rose, Sandalwood, Clary sage, Citrus oils.

Juniper (Juniperus Comninis): Fresh pine-needle aroma. It energizes, relieves exhaustion, cures inflammation, purifies and tones body, improves mental clarity, enhances memory, lessens fluid retention, disinfecting effect, cures cellulits and cystitis (frequent urination), strengthens urinary tract, relieves infection and gout when blended with Vetiver, Sandalwood, Cedarwood, Cypress, Pine, Clary Sage, Lavender, Rosemary.

Lavender (Lavandula Officinalis): Sweet, fresh scent. It balances emotions, relieves stress and tension, cures headache, promotes restful sleep, heels the skin, lowers high blood pressure, helps breathing and cures burns and sunburn when blended with Cedarwood, Clove, Clary Sage, Pine, Gernium, Vetiver, Patecholi.

Lemon (Citrus Limonum): Fresh lemon. It balances nervous system, used as a disinfectant, purifies body, stops bleeding and reduces body temperature when blended with Lavender, Neroli, Fennel, Eucalyptus, Geranium, Camomile, Frankincense, Sandalwood, Rose and Ylang Ylang.

Nature Cure for Allergies

An "allergy" can be described as sensitiveness of the body to substances which can cause mild to violent reactions. Allergic reactions may occur within a few minutes coming in contact with the allergen, or they may be delayed for several hours or even several days. The affected portion of the body is called a shock organ. Common shock organs include the nose, eyes, the skin, chest, intestines, and ears. Symptoms of allergy are recurring headache, migraine, dizziness, irritability, nervousness, depression, neuralgia, sneezing, conjunctivitis, diabetes, eczema, heart burn, hay fever, indigestion, constipation, diarrhea, gastric, ulcer, asthma, overweight, high blood pressure, chest pain, heart attacks, a stuffy or runny nose, breathing problem, swelling of the face and eyes etc.

Causes: An allergic condition may cause from dietetic errors and faulty style of living, irregularities and imbalances due to defective diet and emotional and psychological stress. To treat allery, there are three basic ways: the sources must be identified, once the sources are discovered, they should be avoided and resistance should be built up.

Mud Therapy: Earth was used extensively for remedial purposes in ancient times as well as the middle ages. In modern times, it again has came into prominence as a valuable therapeutic agent. Earth have remarkable effects upon the human body, especially during the night. These effects are described as refreshing, invigorating and vitalising. It is believed that for wounds and skin diseases, application of clay or moistened earth is natural bandage. Going barefooted all day long, except when it is very cold, is also regarded as valuable step towards achieving good health. It is advisable to go entirely barefooted as often as possible, especially on the bare grassy ground. The healing power of earth is very strong as compared to leaves and herbs. This precious gift from the womb of earth not only refreshes, invigorates and revitalises the skin, but also helps in curing chronic inflammation caused by the internal disease; bruises, sprains, boils and sunburn. The cold moisture in the mud packs relaxes the skin pores, draws blood into the surface, relieves congestion and pain besides promoting heat radiation. A mud pack is prepared with clay obtained from about 6 feet below the surface of the earth ensuring that is does not contain impurities such as compose or pebbles. The clay is then made into a smooth paste with warm water, allowed to cool, then spread on a strip of cloth and applied for 15 to 30 minutes.

Mud packs have been found to be a valuable treatment for general weakness, nervous disorders, fever, swelling, eyes and ear troubles, gout, rheumatism, stomach disorders. Mud pack applied to abdomen cures man disorders.

In another mode of treatment, the mud is first ground and then made into a smooth paste mixed with hot water. The paste is then spread on a sheet which in turn is wrapped round the body. A mud pack is followed by a cleansing with warm water followed by a short cold shower. The mud bath is found to tone up the skin by increasing the circulation and energizing the skin tissues. Frequent mud bath improve the complexion, clear spots and patches on the skin and treat skin disease like psoriasis. The duration of the bath should be between 30 to 60 minutes as required.

Enema Therapy: It is known as rectal irrigation. An enema involves the injection of fluid into the rectum. In nature cure treatment, only lukewarm water with or without lime juice is used for cleaning the bowels. An hot water enema is beneficial in relieving irritation due to inflammation of the rectum and painful hemorrhoids. It also benefits women in leucorrhoea (white discharges).

An enema with warm water 1 to 1.5 litres should be taken daily when you are on a diet of fruits or are fasting. If you do not take an enema, there is no benefit from fasting or living on fruits alone. Such enema can help when constipation is very severe. The following points should be kept in mind:

1. Lie down on a hard bed; the foot of the bed must be four inches higher than the head. You can take the enema while lying on the floor, but in that case buttocks should be higher than the rest of body in order to facilitate the introduction of the liquid through the rectum.
2. The vessel containing hot water for the enema should be suspended at a height of three feet from the body. The nozzle should be introduced in the rectum to allow the water to go in.
3. Facilitate the introduction of the enema into the rectum.
4. Let the water go into the rectum, retain it for two to three minutes before going to the toilet.
5. Do not strain at the stools after an enema. Straining will not help clean the bowels as they should be cleaned.

In the case of a enema about 250 millilitres of cold water should be introduced into the intestines and retained for five to ten minutes. Cold water enervates the intestine and gives it tone. An enema can be taken daily and even twice in the day. But prefer to take enema at night before retiring.

Whether the enema water is loss in quantity or not, let the water come out on its own. Do not strain, nor be in a hurry. In the beginning you might have to spend up to 30 minutes in the toilet after taking enema.

Genitals Cleaning: Genital bath is very essential for the cleanliness of genital organs. Keep a stool in the tub. If a stool is not readily available keep four bricks, and sit on them. The water level in the tub should be one inch above the stool. The water should be cold during summer.

Take off your clothes and sit on the stool. Take a piece of cloth, dip it in water and gently rub your abdomen with it for two minutes. Then take hold of the foreskin of your penis in two fingers and rub it lightly with a soft piece of cloth dipping cold water often. This can be continued for ten minutes. After the rubbing of the foreskin is completed, rub the entire spine with a wet towel for two minutes. You can take hold of the wet towel in two hands and move it up and down on your spine.

Women should rub their abdomen. They should take a piece of soft cloth, pull up the lips of the vagina and rub them slowly. And in the end they should also rub the spine as above. No hip bath or genitals bath should be taken at the time of menstruation.

Useful Mud Techniques: The following techniques should be applied.

Bare-foot Walking on the Earth: The earth has magnetic power which stimulates the nerves of entire body. Start with five minutes, then gradually increase the duration up to 30 minutes at the clean hygienic pollution free area. The technique is useful for treating high blood pressure, heart disease, depression and mental tension.

Sleeping on the Earth: Make a sand bed of size 6 feet length, 3 feet thick. Sleeping on mud sand bed for 4 hours equalize 8 hours sleep on the bed. Make sure to remove clothes before lying on sand bed. This will help for treating mental tension, abdomen/body pain, skin diseases, epilepsy, tiredness, hypertension (high blood pressure), heart disease, cancer, anaemia and diabetes.

Sandsun Bath: Make a sand bed in open. Leave for two hours to absorb sun rays. Remove clothes and lie on the bed between 12 noon to 3 p.m. Drink a glass of lime water before sunbathing. Keep a wet towel on the head. Take bath atleast four hours after the meal. The duration of bath should vary between 15-30 minutes. Do not drink water upto 45 minutes and food upto 90 minutes after bath. This is beneficial for curing skin diseases (leducoderma, eczema, varicose veins), myopathy, polyneuritis, inflammation of nerves, diabetes, rheumatism, sleeplessness, polio, paralysis, obesity and venereal diseases e. g. syphilis and gonorrhea.

Mud Sand Bath: Remove clothes and rub mud/sand (in ration of 60:40) on abdomen, breasts, legs, arms and other parts of the body. Have light exercise or walking before bath and rub the body with dry towel to produce heat. Do not have meal for four hours prior to taking bath. Massage at night with coconut or 'arandi' or 'mahua' oil or desi ghee. This will help for body itch, side effect of antibiotics/allopathic medicines, snake bite, high blood pressure, pregnancy, anaemia, heart disease, depression, habit of drinking, body odour and skin disorders e.g., leucoderma, pityriasis, urticaria (shitapitta) and eczema.

Multani-mitti Pack on the Body: Keep multani-mitti (fuller's earth) and water in iron or metallic utensil for 12 hours. Dry massage the body. Apply 1 cm thick pack on the whole body. Have sun bath for 15-30 minutes and rinse off with boiled water. Now massage with coconut oil mixed with lime juice. This technique cures skin diseases such as swelling, sweating, body odour, eczema, dermatitis, leucoderms, burns, urticaria and anaemia.

Mud Bandage: It is beneficial treatment if applied on:

- **The head**: Cure headache, hypertension, high fever sleeplessness and mental tension.
- **On the Spinal Cord and Genital Area:** Has beneficial effect on superior psychic centre and strengthen the nerve system of brain. Cures side effect of antibiotics,

mental tension, anaemia, pregnancy disorders, impotency (when applied bandage on male organs), frigidity (among women) and obesity.

- **On the Eyes:** Has beneficial effect on weak eyesight, watery eyes, glucoma and puffy eyes. To prepare an eye-lotion, mix 25 gms pure honey with 50 ml pure rose water and few drops of lime juice. Put three drops of the eye lotion in each eye in the morning.
- **On the Ears:** Cures pus discharge, inflammation, pain if the mud pack is applied around ears. In case of severe condition, mix neem water or potassium permanganate or epsom salt in the mud.
- **On the Breasts:** Rub with dry towel to stimulate the blood circulation in breast muscles. Apply mud bandage for not more than 15 minutes. It helps to cure respiratory disorders e.g. bronchitis, lungs disorders and tuberculosis.
- **On Abdomen and Waistline:** It is beneficial in curing kidney problems, dysentery, uterus disorders and menstruation problems.
- **On Female Sex Organs:** It is beneficial in the treatment of gynecological disorders. The prominent disorders are connected with menstruation (scanty and painful discharge, profuse bleeding, irregular periods), vaginal discharge of white liquid laced with pus (leucorrhoea or whites), diseases connected with pregnancy and childbirth, inflammation of prostate glands, spotting blood in the urine, itching at vaginal area.

Massage Therapy: Massage is one of the oldest and most useful natural methods of physical treatment. When done properly, the skin becomes flexible and attractive. To master the technique, a thorough knowledge of anatomy of the body and considerable practice in performing the various movements is required by means of the hands or with the aid of mechanical or electrical appliances: such as therapeutic lamps, high frequency facial steamers and vibra-massagers to certain areas of the body, mainly the face, neck, shoulders, the upper chest, back, hands, arms and the scalp. Hands when massaging should be kept soft by the use of creams, oils and lotions to prevent damage to the tissues. The nails should be short and smoothen to prevent any scratching on the skin. The wrist and the fingers should be flexible and the palms firm, warm and dry. Massage should not be done in case of having a weak heart, high blood pressure, inflamed and swollen joints, glandular swelling, abrasion of the skin, broken capillaries of the skin and a skin disease.

A massage improves, develops and tones up the muscular tissues, beautifies the skin and preserves its suppleness. By the action of the hands and fingers the organic waste products can be driven into the blood stream and eliminated. Progressive massage gives the body a chance to free itself from toxic matter, an elegance and good health. An improper massage causes discomfort and pain.

Massage should be done preferably in the morning, after the toilet routine. If you do not have time in the morning, massage at night before going to bed. It should last for 20 to 30 minutes and each area should be massaged for two to five minutes covering the neck, the arms, the legs, the shoulders, the back and the buttocks, the hips and abdomen.

For slimming massage and anti-cellulites, use appropriate creams available in the market. Massage with oil once a week makes the skin supple.

End the massage by taking an alternately hot and cold shower and a friction rub with a coarse towel or wash cloth. Wrinkles are the first sign of ageing and it is an alarming signal. Whether you have lumpy, flabby, withered or sallow skin and wrinkles, your face can regain the appearance of youth under the action of your fingers. Regular daily massage prevents wrinkles on the forehead, temples, eyes, nose, cheeks, mouth and chin.

To ensure good results, observe the following precautions:

- protect your hair with a bandeau and wash your hands.
- Cosmetics clog the skin pores. Remove your make up.
- If skin is oily, use ordinary complexion milk with pH acid.
- If skin is dry, use cleansing milk with witch-hazel base.
- If your skin is dehydrated, use a moisturizing lotion to avoid herpes and wrinkles.
- If skin is too moist, use an astringent lotion to clear pale and puffy look.
- Apply vitamin cream to your face before starting massage. Use a slimming cream if your facial features have a tendency to plumpness.

Basic Manipulations in Facial Massage: These are stroking (effleurage), kneading (petrissage), friction (deep rubbing), percussion (tapotement) and vibrating (shaking). Massage movements are basically of two types Relaxing and Toning. Relaxing movements are slow and soothing whereas Toning movements are rapid and energetic.

- **Stroking Movement**: Consists of running hand very lightly with palms of the hands and pads of the fingers having complete contact with the skin upwards, never downwards. This movement is applied to the forehead, face, scalp, back, shoulders, neck, chest, arms and hands leaving a soothing and relaxing effects which warms, increases blood circulation and soothes the nervous system.
- **Kneading Movement**: Consists of light but firm and deeper movement which clears the waste matter from the muscles, activates the nutrition of the tissues, removes fatigue and increase nervous and muscular energy. This movement gives deeper stimulates and improves the circulation. This movement is good for the chin and the cheeks.

- **Friction Movement**: Employed with fingers and palms over the underlying structures of the skin—this movement leaves influence on the circulation and glandular activity of the skin. Friction movements are usually employed on the scalp, the face and the neck.
- **Percussion Movement**: Leaves a stimulating effect, creates an even force over the treated area on the skin done briskly with the finger-tips. The movement increases blood supply, soothes nerves and strengthens muscles.
- **Vibrating Movement**: It is achieved by rapidly shaking vibrating and pressing with hand or fingers on the body. This movement stimulates circulation, glandular activity and nervous plexuses.

You must Know That: Cottonseed oil is most commonly used for massaging. Butter is used for filling out cheeks, the neck and also for breast enlargement. Oil should not be used by persons with excessive body hair. The oil should be washed off completely after massage. Body massage may be done for 40-45 minutes. It is, however, not recommended in serious inflammatory cases of the joints and infectious diseases which cause formation of pus which may spread the pus to the entire system. In these cases, affected part should first be bathed with hot water for 15 to 30 minutes, then massage should be done for a few minutes.

Avoid deep pressure on swollen nerves, for it will increase the inflammation. Sleeplessness can be cured by slow and gentle massage on the spine and back. Abdominal massage is beneficial in constipation. It stimulates and tones up abdomen muscles. Abdominal massage should not be done in hernia, inflammation of the uterus, bladder, ovaries and fallopian tubes, kidneystones, ulcers of the stomach and intestines, and pregnancy. Avoid abdominal massage after heavy meal. The bladder should be emptied before the massage. Persons with hypertension should also avoid abdominal massage. Chest massage strengthens the chest muscles, increases circulation and tones up the nervous system of the chest, heart and lungs. Massage of the back stimulates the nerves and circulation for treating backache, rheumatic afflictions of the back muscles and for soothing the nervous system.

Physiological Effects of Massage: To obtain proper results from a scalp or facial massage, one must have a thorough knowledge of all the structures involved-the muscles, the nerves and the blood vessels which have a pressure point and a skilful massage influence the structure and function of the body. On these pressure point massage activates circulation, secretion, nutrition and excretion of the skin. The frequency of massage depends upon the age and condition to be treated but in general a weekly massage is recommended. A facial or scalp massage nourishes the skin and its structures, reduce fat cells in the sub-cutaneous tissues, render skin soft and flexible, increase circulation of the blood, stimulate activity of the skin glands, strengthen muscle fibre, refresh (and soothe) nerves and relieve pain.

Remember when indulging in a facial massage try to relax and speak softly or as far as possible keep silent, maintain utmost cleanliness and quiet atmosphere, warm hands before touching the skin and finger-nails should not be too long or pointed. You must observe the following:

- All movements must be made in the direction of the lymphatic circulation—towards the heart.
- When massaging, the arms or the legs movement must go upwards from extremities towards trunk.
- For leg massage, keep the body relaxed, raised which help circulation of blood.
- Do not massage if you are suffering from any infectious disease, fever, heart ailment and after the seventh month of pregnancy.

- Consult doctor, if you suffer from vascular lesions, varicose veins or haemophillia, dermatitis, mycosis, large ovarian cysts, stone in kidney, hernia, recent bone fractures or dislocations.

Reflux Therapy: It has succeeded in several areas of disorder in which no medicine is required. The treatment is simply done through the massage of the foot and helps reducing obesity and extra accumulation of fat on the body, disorders of heart, liver, kidney, stomach, epilepsy, spinal pains, arthritis, stomotitis etc. It is a boon to women suffering from urinary infections, menstrual flow, leucorrhoea, inflammation of reproductive system due to frequent abortions. There are about 75,000 nerve endings in a feet and the congestion in the body builds from the feet. The feet is a mirror image of the body which directly relate to the different organs. By massaging the relevant spots for few minutes every day, symptoms of relief will be visible within a week or so. Regular massaging of feet has a miraculous effect on the face and clears muddy, dull looking skin and dark circles around the eyes. The left feet can help in tackling the malfunctioning of the heart and spleen, whereas the right feet for malfunctioning of liver. For tackling the disorders of stomach, kidney, spine, intestines, eyes, ears-both the feet are massaged simultaneously.

Hormones Therapy: There is a relationship between beauty and hormones. Hormones are produced by the organs in the system of a human body. Lack of hormones or excess of hormones in the body can prove disastrous. Hormones are of various types, but the ones which are associated with beauty are **androgens, estrogens, thyroids, steroids, insulin and sex hormones.** Androgens are basically male hormones. Excessive secretion of androgens, in women produce excessive secretion of sebum which would cause acne, hair loss, stress and mental tension. The imbalance of hormones may be balanced by taking estrogen pills. Estrogens are normally female hormones produced by the ovaries. They help to cure acne and pimples and lead to gain in weight. These hormones benefit the skin by retarding wrinkles, and making it clear and shiny. Estrogen pills are essential for women after the age of 40. Stop taking pills if you suffer from high blood pressure and may harm the skin causing pigmentation and lesions. The shortage of thyroids hormones in the body make skin dry and wrinkled. The excessive Steroids hormones in the body cause infections, pigmentation and acne on the skin. The deficiency of Insulin hormones harm the complexion and cause skin fungus, bacterial infection and itching. Sex hormones: male sex hormones encourage growth of hair on the skin of body where as female sex hormones encourage growth of hair on the scalp.

Herbal Cosmetic Therapy: A balance diet, regular exercise, good night's sleep, satisfying work and relationships and quality are the natural aids to beauty which can help a woman make the most of her looks. Many of the ingredients may even be found in your kitchen. Here are some creams, lotions, face-packs and shampoos that can be made at home by natural ways:

Moisturizer: Suitable for face and hands, a simply mixing equal quantities of glycerin and rose water has been a favourite moisturizer for many years. Increase the quantity of glycerin in case of an excessive dry skin.

Facial Cleansing Cream: Collect 6 tablespoons of beeswax. Heat gently with 450 ml of liquid paraffin on low heat until melted. Allow to cool to 50ºC. Separately heat 300 ml of water, when both are hot at the same temperature, slowly add water to the wax and oil mixture, stirring continuously. Leave to cool until it begins to solidify.

Cold Cream: Pure aloe vera gel give a pleasant texture to cleansing and moisturizing lotion.

Facial Toning Lotion: Contains sage to tighten the skin, close the pores and soothe any spots of inflammation.

Use the lotion after cleansing the skin and before applying any moisturiser. To make the lotion, place three tablespoons of dried sage or 6 of the fresh herb in a clean jar, and pour on it 150 ml of vodka (liquor). After a week, strain off and discard the sage, replacing it with a new measure of the herb and leaving it for another week. Finally, strain the liquid into a clean bottle. Add four or five drops of tincture of benzoin. Screw the lid and shake well. Add 2-3 tablespoons of witch hazel to strengthen the mixture.

Skin refresher: Pawpaw (papaya) fruit contains enzymes that help to remove dead skin, leaving the face fresh and clean. Apply pulped fruit all over the face, leave for a few minutes and then wipe off. Splash with cold water and apply moisturiser.

Facial Masks: These will cleanse and tone the skin, drawing out impurities and soothing sore or inflamed spots. Oatmeal and ground almonds are good all-purpose dry bases, suitable for any skin type.

Herbal Shampoos that Heal the Natural Ways: Choose the right herbs for your hair type when making this gentle shampoo. Use **sage** to condition and enhance the dark hair**, camomile** to lighten and soften fair hair, **mullein** to intensify blonde highlights, **parsley** to thicken and enrich its colour, **southernwoods** to stimulate hair growth, **burdock root** and **nettle** to control dandruff, **kelp** or **yarrow** to encourage growth and check hair loss. **Rosemary** helps in condition the hair.

Egg and Oil Conditioner: Beat together an egg, 2 teaspoons of lemon juice and 1 teaspoon of honey. Heat until creamy, stirring continuously. Remove from heat and when cool slowly mix in 3 tablespoons of safflower or other vegetable oil into which stirr two or three drops of rosemary essential oil.

3

Hydrotherapy-Curing with Bath Treatment

The nature cure system is readjust of the human system from abnormal to normal condition and functioning by the constructive principles of nature. Such methods remove the accumulation of toxic matter and poisons from the system without harming the vital organs of the body. Nature Care stimulates the organs of elimination and purification to better functioning. To cure disease, the first and foremost requirement is to regulate the diet. To get rid of accumulated toxins and restore the equilibrium of the system exclude acid-forming foods including proteins, starches and fats. Continue the diet to fresh fruits which will disinfect the stomach and alimentary canal. If the body is overloaded with morbid matter, a complete fast for a few days may be necessary for the elimination of toxins, fruit juice may, however, be taken during a fast. Do not eat when you are sick, stick to a light diet preferably fresh fruits. Wait for the return of the usual healthy appetite. Loss of appetite is nature's warning to avoid burden on the digestive organs. Alkaline foods such as raw vegetables and sprouted whole grain cereals may be added after a week of a fruit-only diet.

Another important factor in the cure of disease by Naturopathy is to stimulate the vitality of the body using water in various ways and at varying temperatures in the form of packs or baths. The application of cold water to the abdomen—the seat of most diseases and to the sexual organs with the help of cold sitting hip bath lowers body heat and stimulates the nervous system. Hydrotherapy offers a simple natural method of abating fevers and reducing pain and inflammation without any harmful side-effects in the form of wet packs. On the other hand, application of warm water leaves a relaxing effect. Natural methods useful in the cure of diseases are steam and sunbath, exercise and massage. Steam and sunbath revive dead skin and help maintain it in a normal condition. Exercise, especially yogic 'asanas', promote inner health and harmony, and eliminate tension: physical, mental and emotional. Massage tones up the nervous system and quickens blood circulation and the metabolic process. Thus a well balanced diet, sufficient yogic exercise, the observation of the other laws of well-being such as fresh air, plenty of sunlight, pure drinking water, scrupulous cleanliness, adequate rest and right mental attitude can ensure proper health and prevent disease/ disorders as well as tension, depression and fatigue.

Mayur Asana, Setubandha Sarvang Asana, Sirsh Asana, Salamba Sirsh Asana, Viparitakarani, Shav Asana, Suptavajra Asana, Ardha Matsyendra Asana, Shlabh Asana are some of very useful yogic asanas for teenagers and adults. Whereas, regular practice of *Urdhva Hasta Asana, Virbhadra Asana, Prasarita Pada-Uttana Asana, Uttana asana and Adho Mukha Shavana Asana* remove tension and fatigue among children. The Nature Cure claims that in acute diseases, water treatment accomplishes all the beneficial effects without any harmful after-effects upon the system. The principal objects in the treatment of acute inflammatory diseases are:

1. To relieve inner congestion and consequent disorders in affected parts of the body.
2. To increase elimination and thus facilitate the removal of morbid materials from the system in the body.

3. To increase the positive electro magnetic energies in the organism of body.
4. To increase oxygen and ozone in the system, and thereby promote oxidation and combustion of effect matter.
5. To keep body temperature below danger point by promoting heat radiation through the skin.

The application of cold packs to the surface of body draws the blood from the congested interior to the skin, relaxes its minute blood vessels, opens the skin pores, and so facilitates the escape of heat from the body. In inflammatory febrile diseases the blood is congested in the inflamed parts, producing inflammation, such as Rubor (redness), Tumour (swelling), Calor (heat) and Dolor (pain). The various applications of water treatment used singly, combined with regular practice of yogic exercise or alternately according to individual conditions produce the best possible results. A cold water enema is helpful in inflammatory conditions of the colon, especially in cases of dysentery, diarrhoea, ulcerative colitis, hemorrhoids and fever. A hot water enema is beneficial in relieving irritation due to inflammation of the rectum and painful hemorrhoids and fever. It also benefits women in leucorrhoea.

Temperature of water you should be familiar with:

Cold: 40 to 60°F (4. 5 to 15. 5°C)

Cool: 60 to 70°F (15. 5 to 21°C)

Tepid: 70 to 90°F (21 to 32°C)

Warm: 90 to 100°F (32 to 38°C)

Hot: 100 to 110°F (38 to 43°C)

Above 110°F temperature, water loses its therapeutic value and is destructive. Remember, any action is always followed by a reaction which is destructive. The same thing happens with cold water. Another important influence of hydrotherapy is its power to increase the electro-magnetic energies in the human body caused by the sudden application of cold water resulting quickening and deepening of respiration, and also by the resulting contrast of the heat within and the cold outside of the body. This, undoubtedly accounts for the tonic effect of the cold water application. Care must be taken not to lower the temperature too much. Hydrotherapy is much more preferable than antipyretics, which lower resistance. Remember that antipyretics lower metabolism and resistance, while hydrotherapy raises metabolism.

Wet Packs: Wet packs may be applied to any part of the body. The different kinds of packs include Full Sheet Pack, Spanish Mantle, Body Pack, Abdominal Pack, Chest Pack, Scotch Pack, Throat pack, T. Pack, Leg pack, Foot pack and Hip pack. Wet packs help to lower temperature, relieve inner congestion, promote elimination, relieve pain and stimulate sluggish circulation. The packs must be changed as soon as they become dry or uncomfortably hot.

The Full Sheet Pack: Consists use of two or three blankets according to the season, the warmth of the room and the temperature of patient. Spread a bed sheet which has been wrung out in cold water around the body. Pick up the blanket and wrap the sheet around the body.

Spanish Mantle: Consists in giving the patient a whole body sponge with cold water or cool spray and then without drying, wrap him up in a dry sheet and covering with plenty of blankets. When the Spanish mantle is removed the body should be sponged off thoroughly.

Cold and Heating Compress: It is an effective means of controlling inflammatory conditions of the liver, spleen, stomach, kidneys, intestines, lungs, brain, pelvic organs and so on. The cold compress soothes dermatitis and inflammations of the eyes. A heating compress consists of three or four folds of linen cloth wrung out in cold water, which is then covered completely with dry flannel or blanket to prevent the circulation of air and help accumulation of body heat. It is applied for several hours as advised by a naturopath. After removing the compress, the skin should be rubbed with a wet cloth and then dried with a towel. An abdominal compress helps all ailments related to the abdominal organs.

Outdoor Bathing and Swimming: It is very invigorating and beneficial. The bathing and swimming should never be extended to a longer period than 20 minutes. If the reaction is good, there will be a feeling of comfort and warmth, a good appetite and sound refreshing sleep.

Foot Bath: Involves standing in cold water up to the ankles for one or two minutes, then dry the feet with a coarse towel, followed by rubbing the feet vigorously with the hands or walking briskly for a few minutes. Another good mode of this therapy is the barefoot walking on the dewy grass or walking on wet pavements or slabs, followed by drying the foot thoroughly and thereafter taking a brisk walk.

Mud and Clay Packs: Have beneficial result because the cool moisture in and under the pack relax the pores of the skin, draw blood to the surface, relieve inner congestion and pain and promote heat radiation and elimination of morbid matter. Mud and clay have the advantage of easy application, capable to retain moisture and coolness much longer than a water pack or compress.

Mud and clay was used extensively for remedial purposes in the ancient times, and with people going back to nature, it's again in the spotlight. The best way to apply clay packs is to take yellow, or still better, blue Potter's clay, Mix it in warm water until it is reduced to a smooth paste. When cold, spread pack over a strip of cloth wide and long enough to cover the part to be treated and then surround the clay bandage until dry. The process of clay bath is similar to mud bath. It is mixed with hot water and reduced to a smooth paste. The bath must be followed by a cleansing warm spray and finished with a quick tonic cold spray.

Hip Bath: It is one of the most useful forms of hydrotherapy. This mode of treatment involves only the hips and the abdominal region below the navel. A special type of tub used for this purpose is filled with warm water in such a way that it covers the hips and reaches up to the navel when the patient sits in it. If a special tub is not available, a common tub may be used. Hip bath is given in cold, hot, neutral and alternate temperatures.

Cold Hip Bath: The water temperature should be 10 to 18ºC. The duration of bath is usually 30 minutes. If the patient feels cold or is very weak, a hot foot immersion should be given with the cold hip bath. Rub abdomen briskly from the navel downward and across the body with a moderately coarse wet cloth. The legs, feet and upper part of the body should remain completely dry during and after the bath. Undertake moderate yogic exercises after the cold hip bath to warm the body. *Ardha-Matsyendra Asana, Dhanur Asana, Pawan Mukta Asana, Ardha Vakra Asana and Mayur Asana* are most suitable yogic exercises for correct digestive system whereas *Hal Asana and Padma Asana* reduce extra flesh from the hips and abdomen. A cold bath is a routine treatment in most diseases and relieves constipation, indigestion, obesity and uterine problems like irregular menstruation, chronic uterine infections, pelvic inflammation, piles, hepatic congestion, chronic congestion of the prostate glands, seminal weakness, impotency, sterility, ovarian displacement, dilation of stomach and colon, diarrhea, dysentery, hemorrhage of the bladder and many problems.

Hot Hip Bath: It is generally taken for eight to 10 minutes at a water temperature of 40 to 45ºC. The bath should start at 40ºC and the temperature should be gradually increased to 45ºC. Remember, no friction should be applied to the abdomen. Before entering the tub, drink a glass of cold water. A cold compress should be placed on the head. A hot hip bath helps to relieve painful menstruation, pain in the pelvic organs, painful urination, inflamed rectum or bladder and painful piles. It also benefits enlarged prostatic gland, painful contractions or spasm of the bladder. A cold shower bath should be taken immediately after the hot hip bath. The bath should be terminated if the patient feels giddy or complains of excessive pain.

Neutral Bath: The temperature of water should be 32 to 36ºC. Avoid friction to the abdomen. The bath should be taken from 20 minutes to an hour. The neutral hip bath helps to relieve all acute and sub-acute inflammatory conditions.

Hot and Cold Hip Bath: It is also known as repulsive hip bath. The temperature in the hot tub should be 40 to 45ºC and in the cold tub 10 to 18ºC. The patient should alternatively sit in the hot tub for five minutes and then in the cold tub for three minutes. The duration of the bath should be from 10 to 20 minutes. The head and neck should be kept cold with a cold compress. The treatment should end with a dash of cold water to the hips. The bath relieves chronic inflammatory conditions of the pelvic viscera such as salpingitis, ovaritis, cellulitis and various neuralgias of the genito-urinary organs.

Spinal Bath: It is an important form of hydrotherapic treatment. This bath provides a soothing effect to the spinal column and thereby influences the central nervous system. Undertake *Ardha Chandra Asana, Setubandha Sarvang Asana* and *Ushtra Asana* yogic exercises after the bath for excellent results. The bath is given in a specially designed tub with its back raised so as to provide proper support to the head. The bath can be administered at cold, neutral and hot temperatures. The water level in the tub should be two inches and the patient should lie in it for three to 10 minutes. The cold spinal bath relieves irritation, fatigue, hypertension, excitement, all nervous disorders such as hysteria, fits, mental disorders, loss of memory and tension. For better results exercise Yog Asanas e.g. *Supta Vajra Asana, Adho Mukha Shavana Asana, Parasarita Pada Uttan Asana* and

Uttana Asana after the bath. The neutral spinal bath is a soothing and sedative treatment and relieves irritation. The duration of this bath should vary from 20 to 30 minutes. The hot spinal bath helps to stimulate the nerves, especially when they are in a depressed state. It also relieves vertebral pain in spondylitis and muscular backache.

Foot Bath: In hot foot bath, keep legs in a tub or bucket filled with hot water at a temperature of 40 to 45ºC. Before taking this bath, have a glass of water and cover the body with a blanket so that no heat or vapour escapes. The head should be protected with a cold compress. The duration of the bath varies from five to 20 minutes. Take a cold shower immediately after the bath. The hot foot bath stimulates the involuntary muscles of the uterus, intestines, bladder and other pelvic and abdominal organs. It also relieves sprains, ankle joint pains, headaches and restore menstruation among women. In case of cold foot bath, place three to four inches of cold water (temperature of 7.2 to 12.7ºC) in a small tub or a bucket. The feet should be completely immersed in the water for one to five minutes applying friction to the feet during the bath by rubbing one feet against the other. A cold bath relieves cerebral congestion and uterine hemorrhage. It helps in the treatment of sprains, strains and inflamed bunions when taken for longer period. Avoid cold bath in cases of inflammatory conditions of the genito-urinary organs, liver and kidneys.

Steam Bath: Also known as Sauna Bath, is a western concept, it is now gaining popularity in India and other eastern countries. It is one of the most important time-tested water treatments which induces perspiration in a most natural way. Many questions arise. Does Sauna Bath helps you to slim down? Is it good or bad for the skin? How long should one stay in the steam? What dress to wear when having Sauna Bath? In what position should you take this bath?

Sauna helps losing a couple of kilograms, but you may put them on again if you eat or drink immediately after the bath. Do not drink anything for at least one hour after having steam bath. Sauna along with yogic exercise and diet can do wonders in reducing weight. Sauna is a place to relax, to lie prone, speechless. In short, to exercise 15 minutes in Sauna is equivalent to running two kilometres. Toxins are eliminated through the skin and people with specific skin problems like acne and dull, lifeless complexion can clear them up with Sauna. Steam bath is also recommended in clearing cellulitis. Before taking bath, drink one or two glasses of cold water and protect the head with a cold towel. The duration of steam bath is generally 10 to 20 minutes or until profuse perspiration takes place. It is suggested to start with sessions of short duration, and then gradually increase the duration as after some practice the body will withstand the heat for longer period. A cold shower should be taken immediately after the bath. Have a 30 minutes rest at the end to attain the body's normal temperature.

The dress worn at the time of Sauna session is generally briefs and bras or swim suit. A bare body will reap more benefit than a covered one. Women generally feel shy, but gradually they overcome their shyness in the nude. Persons taking steam bath are only interested in their own bodies. Do not wear watch and jewellery when taking steam bath. The steam and heat shall damage them badly. To sit up or to lie is another important question that people want to ask. It is said that the heat penetrates more if you sit up. Some people when attending Sauna session lie on their tummies, some on their backs. It is preferred to lie on the back. Saunas are not conductive to hair, so better wrap hair in a towel.

Epsom Salt Bath: Fill the bath tub with about 135 litres of hot water at 40°C. One to 1.5 kg of Epsom salt should be dissolved in this water. Before taking bath, drink a glass of cold water, cover the head with a cold towel and then lie down in the tub completely immersing the trunk, thighs and legs for 15 to 20 minutes. The best time to take bath is just before retiring to bed. This bath is very useful for the skin besides disorders of kidney, sciatica, lumbago, rheumatism, diabetes, neuritis, cold and catarrh.

Sea Water Bath: Cleanses the skin, firms the muscles, stimulates the circulation and tones up the system. Remember that sea water dries the skin and the hair. After having a bath or swim in sea water, wash yourself with fresh water and rub a little almond oil on the skin. When you swim, protect your hair with a water-tight cap.

Tap Water Bath: It can be good for skin, depending on skin type and the hardness or softness of the water. If your skin is extremely dry, washing face in tap water will not be helpful, for the salts and calcium in the water will almost certainly be drying. Use of a water softener (bath salt or oil), when washing, will help to counteract this effect. Beware of using hard water on your face.

Twenty Minutes Luxury Bath: On a holiday, take a twenty minute luxury bath. To take bath, pour scented bath oil or bubble bath in the tub and run the tap. In the morning prefer to take your bath under the shower. Cold water closes the skin pores and helps you shake off early morning sluggishness. While the tap is running, undress and tuck your hair away from your face and neck. Remove face make up, if any, with a cleansing lotion. Take off your bath robe and get into the bath tub, and relax completely for a few minutes. Now apply soap to the upper part of your body. Rub every part except your breasts (in case of women) with the friction mitt. Pay particular attention to your neck. This is usually a neglected area which sometimes becomes gray because of bad circulation. Rubbing with the mitt will help to improve this. Give circulation to your upper arms, elbows and shoulders too and use friction mitt on legs, heels and ankles. Use a bath brush to give the back of your body a thorough scrub and prevent spots. Use an anti-perspirant in the arm-pits. Relax again for at least five minutes before stepping out of the bath. Then towel your body dry by patting and rubbing it very gently. Apply talcum powder on underarms, feet and pubic area with firm, gentle strokes. Rub body lotion or massage cream on the rest of your body. Use both hands to rub over back, bottom, breasts, legs, stomach and arms. After your bath, try to relax for a few minutes.

Be careful when applying cold water to breasts. Only douche the tips of the nipples and do it very quickly. Prolonged washing of the breasts could chill the mammary glands deeply and cause bronchitis. Many women use ice to rub over the tips of the breasts. The intense cold causes a very strong static contraction in the mammary muscles without giving the time to cause a chill.

Here are Few Herbal Baths

(a) **Milk Bath:** Cleopatra bathed in ass' milk and so also did Poppaaca, the wife of Nero. These days, it is not possible to afford milk for bathing. Here is an alternate process for similar results. Add a handful of powdered milk to the bath water.

(b) **Soft-Water Bath:** Use of rainy water is very beneficial. If you cannot get rain water, soften the bath water by simply adding a little sodium sesqui carbonate.

(c) **Vinegar Bath:** It is very useful for itchy or dry skin. Add a cup of vinegar to the bath water.

(d) **Oatmeal or Bran Bath:** Put one tablespoon of oatmeal in bath. Oatmeal and bran contain oils and vegetable hormones, which soothe and soften the skin.

(e) **Honey Bath:** To give the body skin feeling smooth and satiny, add a teaspoon of honey to your bath water.

(f) **Starchy Bath:** Mix a few tablespoons of laundry starch and a teaspoon of glycerin to your bath water. It will leave your skin beautifully smooth, tight and soft.

(g) **Herb Bath:** Lavender, hyssop, mint, borage, yarrow,

rosemary, balm or camomile are useful herbs for the skin used in bath water either separately or in a mixture.

(h) **Salt Bath:** Mix two cups ordinary washing soda, two tablespoons potassium carbonate and four to five drops of Aromatic oil (lavender or pine oil). Use about a tablespoon of this mixture in a bucket of bath water.

(i) **Oil Bath:** Mix a little quantity of almond or olive or sunflower oil to bath water. Baby oil or mineral oil is not suitable as it cannot be absorbed by the skin.

(j) **Bubble Bath:** Mix and beat one egg, 1/2 cup shampoo and one teaspoon gelatine. Add the mixture to bath water when the tap is running.

(k) **Milk and Honey Bath:** Collect ingredients such as 2 eggs, 1/4 cup each almond and sunflower oil, 1/2 cup olive oil, 1 teaspoon honey, 2 teaspoons washing detergent, 1/4 cup vodka, 1/2 cup milk and few drop perfume.

Completely blend the eggs, honey and oils together. Now add to it the detergent. Continue beating and add Vodka. Add to it milk which will make the oil slightly thinner and luxurious. Finally, add perfume. This bath oil when mixed to bath water leaves the skin feeling smooth, satiny and thoroughly pampered.

Precautions While Taking Therapeutic Bath?

- Avoid bath within three hours after a meal and one hour before it. Avoid hip bath and foot bath two hours after a meal.
- Use clean and pure water for bathing. For desired effects, temperature of water and the duration of bath should be strictly observed.
- Women should not take any of the baths during menstruation. Pregnants can take only hip bath till the completion of third month.

Sun Bath: Clears the skin of acne, heals mild infections, cleanses oily skins, gives a lovely tan and revives the whole body. On the other hand, hot sunbath can wither a dry skin, burn a delicate one, distend the veins, and cause burns and sunstroke. Sun bathing must be progressive, five minutes on the first day, ten minutes on the second and fifteen minutes on the third day. Never expose yourself continuously to the strong rays of the sun for more than half an hour at a time. To enjoy the beneficent effects of the sun is to play, walk or swim in sunlight. Do not use eau-de-cologne, perfume, deodorants or wear heavy make-up while going out in sun, these can cause brown marks and irritation to the skin.

Cold: Makes your cheeks dry, cracks the skin and hinders the blood circulation. Protect your skin with a thick coating of cream. Even oily skin must be lubricated during winter. Avoid going abruptly from the cold outside to a hot air-conditioned room, which can cause blood vessels under the skin and cause a blotchy complexion.

Wind: The wind stimulates the circulation and can be a tonic to the system, but it dries the skin, especially during winters or summers. Protect your facial skin with cold cream.

Curative Power of Sun Charged Water: Acute as well as chronic diseases such as headache, blood pressure, anaemia, gout, paralysis, acidity, abnormal palpitation and convulsions, cough, asthma, TB, ENT disorders, meningitis, liver disorders brain troubles, hyper acidity, gastritis, dysentery, constipation, piles, diabetes, irregular menses, leucorrhoea, cancer of uterus can be cured by white water treatment.

Take about four glasses of white charged water (1 litre) at a time early morning. Nothing should be taken within one hour of taking this water. Do not take water for two hours after breakfast and lunch. Start with two glasses of water and gradually increase the amount to four glasses.

Different types of diseases can be cured with this method within the time limit given below:

Disease		Curative Period
Cancer	:	6 months
Constipation	:	10 days
Diabetes	:	1 month
Gastric trouble	:	10 days
Hypertension	:	1 month
Tuberculosis	:	1 month

Following precautions are needed for the treatments:

- Store white charge water in a copper container or earthen pot.
- Water should be taken only before sunrise.
- Avoid eating oil spices, chilies, condiments, etc.
- After taking this drink, one should not lie on bed.
- Wash hands and feet before taking the drink.
- Store sun charged water on the previous night in silver, copper, brass, stone, glass or clay container.

Note: In case of cloudy weather it is difficult to charge water in the absence of sun, fresh collected tap water may be used within 15 to 20 minutes. Avoid drinking water in case of diseases like dropsy, jaundice, rheumatism, rheumatic fever etc. Sun charged water or boiled water has no adverse effect on the health.

Turkish Bath: This is a very old procedure, dating back to the time of the Romans. In this bath, the air is heated in a chamber especially fitted up for its application, the essential features of which are: dressing-rooms, a warm room having (temperature 43°C to 54°C) or hot room having (temperature 65.5°C to 76.5°C), a shampoo room having a douche apparatus, a plunge bath, and a cooling room. The air of the rooms may be heated by steam coils or by electric currents or hot air or indirect radiation. Turkish bath rooms are provided with steam-coils or pipes.

The turkish bath is similar to the hot air bath, but differs as the whole body is given friction, kneading of the muscles, and shampooing. Before entering the bath, the patient should drink hot or cold water, according to his preference. 3 to 4 glasses of water should be taken at intervals during the bath. During the first 10 to 15 minutes, the patient is frequently rubbed for one or two minutes. To induce perspiration, apply a hot foot bath or a hot fomentation to the spine. When the patient begins to perspire, he should enter the hot room from hot room the patient goes to the shampoo room. Rubbings and stroking are continued until the skin is smooth and polished. These movements are simple firm pressure with the hands, rapid to-and-fro movements on the chest and abdomen. Finally stroking movements are applied.

The physiological effects of the Turkish bath are not similar to those of the hot air bath. It is seen patients lose 800 gms or more in a single bath of an hour's duration. The turkish bath may be usefully employed in the majority of chronic disorders. The Turkish bath should not be employed in cases of skin disease accompanied by eruptions, on account of the excessive congestion of the skin. It must be avoided in most cases of organic disease of the heart, kidneys and diabetes. Avoid the overuse of Turkish bath.

The Graduated Bath: It is a form of the full bath especially used for the treatment of fevers. The initial temperature of the bath should be one or two degrees below the temperature of the patient. The patient should be continuously rubbed to produce chilly sensations in fevers the bath is administered every three hours. Remember persons suffering from heart disease should not be administered a very cold bath. The physiological effect of the graduated bath is to reduce the body temperature. To increase vital resistance or to energies the heart a cold friction, a cold towel rub, rubbing wet sheet or ice-bag is recommended.

Cold Friction: Cold friction is a procedure which involves the application of a series of partial wet rubbings to the surface of the body, one part after another being taken in systematic order until the whole surface has been brought into vigorous reaction with the help of cold water or ice water. The patient should be undressed, and made to lie upon bed wrapped in a turkish sheet. First of all the head, face, and neck should be wet with cold water. Then dip the mitt into the cold water and rub the surface of the patient's body rapidly until it reddens. Start with the front of the trunk, after that in succession the legs, the back, the hips, back of the legs, and lastly the feet. The soles of the feet should not be rubbed. The act of rubbing the surface produces mechanical effect similar to those from the impact of water under pressure as in the douche. Therapeutic Applications include powerfully stimulation, the cerebral functions and tonic applications. Cold friction is employed in cases of anaemia, chlorosis tuberculosis and cardiac dropsy. Cold friction is also beneficial in case of typhoid fever, diabetics, dicrotic pulse, subnormal temperature, pregnancy puerperal fever, chronic dysentery, malarial fever, coma from any cause, whooping cough, yellow fever, plague, dengue, influenza, lithemia, leprosy, emaciation, scurvy, rickets, purpura, anorexia, hypopepsia, intestinal catarrh, chronic nephritis, hysteria, neurasthenia, migraine, paralysis agitans and other drug habits. Cold friction should be employed every two or three hours or at least two or three times a day.

Hot Air Bath: Consist in exposure of the entire body with the exception of the head to a superheated atmosphere. The patient is undressed and placed upon a stool or a bed in a cabinet. The air in cabinet is gradually heated to the desired temperature from 48°C to 93°C. However, a temperature of 60°C to 82°C is sufficient to produce profuse perspiration. Perspiration should be encouraged by making the patient drink a glass of water before going into the bath, and if possible, one or two more during the bath. It may precede a cold douche, a cold wet pack, a cold immersion, a cold sponge, or a wet sheet rub. If there is a tendency to cerebral congestion during the bath, a towel saturated with cold water or an ice collar may be place around the neck. Care must be taken in administering hot-air bath to avoid sudden and excessive applications of heat to the skin, which will result in dilatation of the surface blood vessels. The purpose of the cold application following the hot bath is, to increase the tonus of blood vessels, to energize the nerve centres, and to change the condition of passive congestion of the skin. The first physiological effects of the hot-air bath is to heat the skin and body and to raise temperature of blood to a sufficient degree to cause perspiration. The skin becomes red. High temperature must never be employed in cardiac cases. The hot air bath should be avoided in case of skin disorders, cardiac weakness, in the febrile conditions, in diabetes and in advanced cases of nephritis.

Electric Therapy: Electricity is a form of energy, which when in motion, produces magnetic, chemical or heat effects. The beneficial effects of electricity have been recognized to be of great value in cosmetology and very useful for skin care. The electric current is passed through wires, which is composed of twisted, fine metal threads covered with insulator. For using electricity for skin care, you should know about the different currents that can be used and their various uses. There are four types of current: Galvanic, Faradic, Sinusoidal and High Frequency.

Galvanic Current: It is a constant and direct current having opposite poles i.e. positive pole (anode) and negative pole (cathode). Positive pole has acid reaction, soothes nerves, decreases blood supply and hardens tissues. On the other hand, negative pole has alkaline reaction, irritates nerves, increases blood supply and softens tissues. Positive pole (anode) may be used for the conditions such as to make flabby skin and tissues firmer, to close the skin pores after finishing a facial treatment, to decrease redness as in mild-acne, to prevent inflammation after come-done treatment, electrolysis and to force astringent lotions into the skin.

Negative Pole (cathode) may be used for the conditions such as to remove superfluous hair by electrolysis, to stimulate the circulation and nutrition of dry, pale skin and scalp and to force bleaching solution into the skin.

Faradic Current: It is an alternating and interrupted current capable of producing a mechanical reaction, without a chemical effect. When the faradic current is applied to the body, the muscles are toned, and circulation of blood improves. It stimulates hair growth and increases glandular activity. Faradic current may be used during scalp and facial manipulations. Do not use Faradic Current if it causes pain or discomfort, you have high blood pressure and broken capillaries and suffer a pustular condition of the skin.

Sinusoidal Current: It is an alternating current having advantages such as it has greater stimulation and deeper penetrating effect, soothes the nerves and penetrates into the deeper muscle tissue. Do not use sinusoidal current if the face is very flushed, you have broken capillaries on the skin, you have any pustular condition of the skin, you suffer from high blood pressure and the duration is more than 15 minutes.

High Frequency Current: It is very useful for both scalp and facial treatments. The Electrodes of high frequency are made of glass or metal. As the current passes through the glass electrodes, tiny violet sparks are emitted. The treatment should be started with a mild current and then gradually increased. The duration of high frequency current depends upon the condition to be treated and for a general facial a duration of about five minutes is adequate. A high frequency current is useful to stimulate the circulation of the blood, increase glandular activity, treat falling hair and itchy scalp and cure excessively oily or dry skin and scalp.

4

Nature Care for Digestive Disorders

A healthy body is beautiful. A fat surplus of 8 to 15 per cent, over the normal weight, must be considered as overweight. Beyond that, it is obesity. Over 30 per cent, it is extreme obesity. Heredity factor, habit of overeating, ageing factor, poor functioning of the system, nervous factor, sedentary life causing constipation and glandular system causing over-secretion by part of the sub renal glands are some of the causes of overweight.

There are three categories of overweight: fatty overweight, watery overweight and cellulites.

Fatty overweight is really 'fat and muscle' uniformly spread and is more usual in men. It is often more noticeable over the upper half of the body-head, neck, arms and trunk. Watery overweight does not affect the muscles is most usual over the lower half of the body and is common in women. Cellulites is a form of infiltration rather than overweight.

Warning Signals

- The skirt belt or jean gets a little tight.
- There is strain on jacket buttons.
- The face starts growing round.
- The skin gets puffy.

- The skin loses its firm and taut.
- Shoulders get plump and the hollows over the collar-bones.
- Fat overhangs the hips and the waist will disappear.
- The buttocks enlarge.
- The girdle squeezes the flesh, the roll of which will swell out above and below it.
- The neck thickens and lose its normal contour.
- A double chin under the nape of the neck follows.
- Breasts sag down to the stomach, the stomach droops over the pubis and the pubis swells modestly over the genital organs.

Being over-weight not only affects one's looks and figure, but also damages one's health. Being over-weight causes:

(a) *Circulation Problem*: The obese persons with slight exertion, get palpitations, experience pain in the heart. The heart gets tired resulting in heart troubles. There is always a possibility of high blood pressure and diabetes or gout (gathia).

(b) *Psychological and Nervous Troubles*: Causing irritation, tiredness, nervousness, athletic and lethargic atmosphere among obese.

(c) *Digestive Problems*: Cause dilation of stomach, inflammation, spasma of intestines, congestion of liver and digestive upsets.

(d) *Genital Disorders*: The infiltration of fat into the nervous and glandular tissues which control sexual appetite cause impotence.

Girls between the age of 14 and 18 tend to put on excess weight, largely because their bodies are undergoing natural changes around this time. Women, face this problem after their first baby. Obesity is disastrous for women looking for a career. It becomes a real mental burden for those afflicted with it. Even if the problem does not cause danger to physical health, its psychological effect can be far more damaging. Remember, slimming can be done without tears by practicing yogic exercises regularly. To maintain a perfect figure, the amount of energy you consume must be equal to the amount of energy you burn.

Over Weight: Obesity has become a worldwide health hazard for majority of people-male and female of every age. There is a difference between obesity and overweight. Overweight is not obesity, but every obese person is overweight. It has been observed that an obese person loses average two to three kgs of weight every month to fight obesity practicing a few selected yogic postures supported by a balanced and proper diet. Recommended exercises to fight over weight include *Surya Namaskar Asana, Manduk Asana, Chakar Asana, Dhanur Asana, Janusir Asana, Janusir Merudanda Asana, Parivrtta Janusir Asana*

(a) **Yoga Postures for Slimming Back:** These are Baddha Kona Asana, Hal Asana, Paschimottan Asana, Padahasta Asana, Shallabh Asana, Virbhadra Asana and Karna Pida Asana.

(b) **Yoga Postures to Relieve Fatness on Hip:** These are Kon Asana, Hal Asana, Mal Asana, Janusir Asana, Vajroli Mudra, Parivratta Asana.

(c) **Yoga Postures to Shed Off Fat Around Stomach, Waist and Trunk:** Supta-Vajra Asana.

(d) **Yoga Postures to Slim Abdomen:** Yog Mudra, Urdhva Prasarita, Pada Asana, Uttan Asana, Paschimottan Asana, Mayur Asana, Shallabh Asana, Uddiyana Bandha.

(e) **Postures for the Slimming of Legs, Knees, Ankles and Thighs:** Meditation, Supta-Vajar Asana, Vakra Asana, Ardh Bhujang Asana, Utthita Asana, Utthita Trikona Asana, Vir bhadra Asana, Ardh Chandra Asana.

(f) **Postures to Trim Arms, Hands and Wrists:** Utthita Padma Asana, Bak Asana, Pas Asana, Janusir Asana, Parvirtta Asana.

(g) **Postures to Relieve Spinal Column Deformities:** Ardha Chandra Asana, Hal Asana, Karna Pida Asana, Setu-bandha Sarvang Asana, Bhujang Asana.

(h) **Postures for Slimming Abdomen:** Kukkuta Asana, Paschimottan Asana, Tri-anga Mukha-Ek-Pada Asana, Dhanur Asana.

(i) **Postures for Slimming Whole Body:** Garuda Asana, Parivratta Trikona Asana.

Calorie-Controlled Diet: Calories are themselves energy units, and all foods contain calories to a greater or lesser degree. A normal everyday diet of a woman who is not pregnant, or who is not engaged in strenuous physical labour requires 2200 to 2300 calories daily to fulfill the needs of a healthy average woman. A normal healthy male person needs approx. 2500 calories in a day. Protein intake should account for about 50 per cent of daily calories consumption with the rest taken up by fresh vegetables, fruits with carbohydrates kept to the minimum. Starchy and foods containing sugar should be minimized as much as possible in favour of protein-rich foods.

Diet Chart Ratio of Calories

Vegetarian Diet	*Non-vegetarian Diet*
Protein: 30%	Protein: 30%
Carbohydrates: 65%	Carbohydrates: 50%
Fat: 5%	Fat: 20%

Normally, a healthy body digests the food within 15 to 20 minutes and converts it into energy. Correct choice of food, the method of cooking, punctuality and regularity of food timings are important for good health.

Ideal Weight

According to an old conventional standard, a man should weigh 2. 5 times as many kilograms as he is inches taller than 3 feet 3 inches. For example, 5 feet 7 inches tall fully dressed man should weigh approximately 74 kgs. This method of calculation will be lesser in case of a woman whose muscular development is considerably less. Apart from exercise, reduce intake of food. What needed is a quantity of diet on the one hand and a quality diet on the other. Cut out fat and alcohol. Reduce carbohydrates to a minimum but retain a sufficient amount of proteins. Normally a healthy food can be digested within 15 to 20 minutes and converts it into energy. Food must contain a balanced quantity of proteins and carbohydrates. A young woman of average height, who is not pregnant, or who is not engaged in hard physical labour, requires approx. 2300 calories a day. One gram protein or carbohydrate gives four calories whereas One gram of fat gives nine calories. Milk, eggs, meat and fish, soyabean, almond, coconut, groundnut etc. are rich sources of protein and give strength to the body. Carbohydrates is found in vegetables, fruits, cereals and helps other food in generating calories. Deficiency of carbohydrates leads to weakness.

Nutrition and Food Therapy: Dr. Benedict Lust (1872-1945) is called the Father of Naturopathy. Nature cure is based on the realization that man is born healthy and strong and that he can stay as such by living in accordance with the laws of nature. Fresh air, sunshine, a proper diet, exercise, scientific relaxation, constructive thinking and the right mental attitude, meditation and yogic pranayama—all play their part in keeping a sound mind in a sound body.

Nature cure believes that disease is an abnormal condition of the body resulting from the violation of the natural laws. Every such violation has repercussions on the human system, in the shape of lowered vitality, irregularities of the blood and lymph and the accumulation of waste matter and toxins. When toxins accumulate, other organs such as the bowels, kidneys, skin and lungs are worst affected. The whole philosophy and practice of nature cure is built on three basic principles. The first and most basic principle of nature cure is the accumulation of waste materials which are removed from the system through the organs of elimination. These are steadily piling up in the body through faulty living habit, such as wrong feeding, improper body care and habits, worry, overwork and excesses of all kinds. The only way to cure disease is to employ methods which will enable the system to throw off these toxic accumulations. The second basic principle of nature cure is that all acute diseases such as fevers, colds, inflammations, digestive disturbances and skin eruptions are nothing more than self-initiated efforts on the part of the body to throw off the accumulated waste materials through harmful methods such as drugs, vaccines, narcotics and gland extracts. The third principle of nature cure is that the body contains an elaborate healing mechanism which has the power to bring about a return to normal condition of health. The power to cure diseases lies within the body itself and not in the hands of the doctor. The modern medical system treats the symptoms and suppresses the disease but does little to ascertain the real cause, Toxic drugs, may suppress or relieve ailments, usually have harmful side-effects. When drugs are used, the patient has to recover twice-once from the illness, and once from the drug. The power to restore health lies not in drugs, but in nature.

Naturopathy: The Drugless Therapy: To cure disease, the first and foremost requirement is to regulate the diet. To get rid of accumulated toxins and restore the equilibrium of the system, it is desirable to completely exclude acid-forming foods including proteins, starches and fats and to confine the diet to fresh fruits which will disinfect the stomach and alimentary canal. If the body is overloaded with morbid matter, a complete fast for a few days may be necessary for the elimination of toxins. Fruit juice may, however, be taken during a fast. A simple rule is: do not eat when you are sick, stick to a light diet of fresh fruits. Wait for the return of the usual healthy appetite. Loss of appetite is Nature's warning that no burden should be placed on the digestive organs. Alkaline foods such as raw vegetables and sprouted whole grain cereals may be added after a week of a fruits-only diet.

Another important factor in the cure of diseases by natural methods is to stimulate the vitality of the body. This can be achieved by using water in various ways and at varying temperatures in the form of packs or baths. The application of cold water, especially to the abdomen, the seat of most diseases, and to the sexual organs, through a cold sitting (hip bath) immediately lowers body heat and stimulates the nervous system. In the form of wet packs, hydrotherapy offers a simple natural method of combating fevers and reducing pain and inflammation, without any harmful side-effects.

Other natural methods useful in the cure of diseases are air and sun baths, exercise and massage. Air and sunbaths revive dead skin and help maintain it in a normal condition. Exercise, especially yogic asanas, promote inner health and harmony and help eliminate all tension: physical, mental and emotional. Massage tones up the nervous system and quickens blood circulation and the metabolic process. Thus a well-balanced diet, sufficient physical exercise, the observation of the other laws of well-being such as fresh air, plenty of sunlight, pure drinking water, scrupulous cleanliness, adequate rest and right mental attitude can ensure proper health and prevent disease.

Recommended Dietary Allowance (RDA): The Recommended Dietary Allowance (RDA), suggested for Indian men and women with a moderate activity level is given here with an explanation of the functions and sources of all the major nutrients usually required by men, working women, lactating mothers and during pregnancy. A woman should consume approximately 1900 to 2200 and men approx 2200 to 2500 kcal/day as daily energy requirement. However, during pregnancy and breast feeding your energy requirements are higher and you will need to consume between 2200 to 2500 kcal/day. These requirements should be supplemented by a balanced combination of carbohydrates, protein, vegetables and fat moderation. The keyword here is quality and not quantity. It's not about how much you eat, but what you eat. The following tips are suggested:

1. All food groups provide energy, which is expressed in technical terms as kilocalories (kcal). You need to provide your body with 2200 to 2500 kcal of Energy per day.
2. Protein (65 gm/day) is required for a good overall growth and development. Pulses, dairy products, Soyabean are an excellent source of vegetarian protein.
3. Calcium (1000 mg/day) is required for the development of bones and teeth. Dairy products (milk, pasteurized cheese, paneer, curds etc.), soyabean products, dark green leafy vegetables and sesame seeds are loaded with calcium.
4. Iron (40mg/day) is an essential component of haemoglobin that supplies oxygen to each cell of the human body, especially red blood cell production. Foods with high iron sources are dried beans, cereals and pulses, dried fruits, dark green leafy vegetables, til, nuts and jaggery.
5. Folic acid (400 mcg/day) is an essential vitamin required especially for women going to conceive and also during the early stage of pregnancy for the growth and development of the foetus throughout the pregnancy and breast feeding. Its deficiency leads to anaemia. Potatoes, vegetables, cereals and pulses, soyabean, nuts and sesame seeds are rich source of Folic Acid.

6. Fat (30 gms Per/day) is essential to enhance energy.
7. Vitamin C (40 mg/day) is necessary to fight against infections and diseases. It provides structure to the bones, cartilage, muscles and blood vessels. Citrus fruits, amla, vegetables and fruits boost up with plenty of vitamin C.
8. Vitamin A (Beta-Carotene 2400 mcg/day) is required for clear vision and healthy skin. Excessive vitamin A leads to toxicity and can be harmful. Maintain Vitamin A level with yellow orange, vegetables (carrot and pumpkin), fruits (mango, papaya and tomatoes), green leafy vegetables and whole milk.
9. Vitamin D is synthesized through sunlight which aids the absorption of calcium in the body.
10. To maintain adequate diet iodine levels in body, use daily diet. Natural sources like Cereals, nuts and oilseeds are rich in Iodine mineral.

Breast Milk

Breast feeding is very important as it helps to build a strong bond between mother and the baby, and is also the best form of nourishment for newborn infant. The quantity and quality of milk produced is not related to the size of breast but is dependent on the amount of fluids you consume. A feeding mother should drink plenty of juices, milk shakes, buttermilk, soups, water etc. Have at least 4 litres of fluid per day. Breast milk is a natural, pure and unadulterated form of nourishment for the child. It provides antibodies to the baby which is why it is superior to formula feeds or cow's milk. Breast feeding nurtures the emotional bonding between the mother and child. The nutritional quality of breast milk is much higher than that of cow's milk or buffalo's milk as it contains more lactose (more sugar), more vitamin A, C and E, fat and iron. Breast feeding women and expectant, mothers require a lot more calories during pregnancy. This is because breast feeding baby will make mother burn 3500 kcal per day. However, the mother consume only 2400 to 2700 kcal per day during the first 6 months of lactation.

Juice Therapy: It is known as juice fasting and is most effective way to restore health and rejuvenate the body. Raw juice therapy is a method of treatment of disease through an exclusive diet of juices of fruits and vegetables. An exclusive diet of raw juices of fruits and vegetables results in much faster recovery from diseases and more effective cleansing and regeneration of the tissues than the fasting on pure water. Drinking alkali-forming fruit and vegetable juices, during fasting increase the healing effect of fasting and elimination of uric acid and other inorganic acids will be accelerated. Sugar in juices strengthen the heart. All juices should be made fresh immediately before drinking. Raw juices from root vegetables may be combined with those of green leafy vegetables, but not with other juices. A glass of water mixed with lemon juice and 20 to 30 grams of honey may be taken first in the morning. Thereafter, the prescribed juice may be taken at three-hourly intervals. The patient should take adequate rest during the raw juice therapy. A proper selection of juices in treating a particular ailment is very essential. Fruit and vegetable juices found beneficial in their treatment are mentioned below:

Disorder	**Suggested Juice**
Acidity:	Grapes, orange, mosambi, lemon, carrot and spinach.
Acne/Pimples:	Grapes, pear, plum, tomato, cucumber, carrot, potato and spinach.
Allergies:	Apricot, grapes, carrot, beet and spinach.
Anaemia:	Apricot, strawberry, red grape, beet, celery and carrot.
Arthritis:	Pineapple, apple, lemon, cucumber, carrot, lettuce and spinach.

Asthma:	Apricot, lemon, pineapple, peach, carrot, radish and celery.
Bronchitis:	Apricot, lemon, pineapple, peach, tomato, carrot, onion and spinach.
Bladder:	Apple, apricot, lemon, cucumber, carrot, parsley and watercress.
Colds:	Lemon, orange, grapefruit, pineapple, carrot, onion and spinach.
Constipation:	Apple, pear, grapes, lemon, carrot, beet, spinach and watercress.
Colitis:	Apple, apricot, pear, peach, pineapple, papaya, carrot and spinach.
Diabetes:	Citrus fruits, carrot, celery, lettuce and spinach.
Diarrhoea:	Papaya, lemon, pineapple, carrot and celery.
Eczema:	Red grapes, carrot, spinach, cucumber and beet.
Epilepsy:	Red grapes, figs, carrot, celery and spinach.
Eye Disorders:	Apricot, tomato, carrot, celery, parsley and spinach.
Gout:	Red sour cherries, pineapple, tomato, cucumber and spinach.
Halitosis:	Apple, grapefruit, lemon, pineapple, tomato, carrot and spinach.
Headache:	Grapes, lemon, carrot, lettuce and spinach.
Heart Disease:	Red grapes, lemon, cucumber, carrot, beet and spinach.
Hypertension:	Grapes, orange, cucumber, carrot and beet.

Insomnia:	Apple, grapes, lemon, lettuce, carrot and celery.
Jaundice:	Lemon, grapes, pear, carrot, celery, spinach and cucumber.
Kidney:	Apple, orange, lemon, cucumber, carrot, parsley and beet.
Lever ailments:	Lemon, papaya, grapes, carrot, tomato, beet and cucumber.
Menstruation:	Grapes, prunes, cherry, spinach, lettuce, turnips and beet.
Menopausal:	Fruits and Vegetables in season.
Neuritis:	Orange, pineapple, apple, carrot and beet.
Obesity:	Lemon, grapefruit, orange, cherry, pineapple, cabbage and carrot.
Piles:	Lemon, orange, papaya, pineapple, turnip and watercress.
Prostrate:	All fruit juices in season, carrot, lettuce and spinach.
Psoriasis:	Grapes, carrot, beet and cucumber.
Rheumatism:	Grapes, orange, lemon, tomato, carrot and spinach.
Stomach Ulcers:	Apricot, grapes, cabbage and carrot.
Sinus Trouble:	Apricot, lemon, tomato, carrot, onion and radish.
Sore Throat:	Apricot, grapes, lemon, pineapple, carrot and parsley.
Tonsillitis:	Apricot, lemon, orange, grapefruit, pineapple, carrot and radish.
Varicose Veins:	Grapes, orange, tomato, beetroot, carrot and watercress.

Natural FOOD Products for health and beauty

Name of Product	*Used Extensively for*
Adrak (Ginger)	Helps digestion, increases appetite, reduces the flatulence resulting from certain foods.
Ajwain (caraway seeds)	Helps in disorders of the liver, stomach and the intestines.
Amla (Emblic)	Source of Vitamin C, falling and premature greying hair and rejuvenates the body.
Papaya (Papita)	Acts as digestive agent. Reduces inflammation of liver and spleen. Cures ringworm and intestinal parasites.
Babchi (Psorales Corylifolia)	Cures leucoderma (white patches on the skin).
Babool (Kikar)	Relieves diarrhoea, prevent threatened abortion, useful in case of cough, asthama and prolapse of the rectum.
Buttermilk	The mask helps to get rid of freckles.
Carrot (Gajar)	Full of vitamins A, B and C. Used as face mask.
Castor oil	Lubricate eyebrows and eyelashes, condition dry hair and aid dry skin.

(Contd.

Name of Product	*Used Extensively for*
Cocoa butter (Coconut oil)	Makes a good hair conditioner. Used as gentle body rub and hand lotion.
Cosmetic Vinegar (Cider)	Keep the skin around eyes smooth and wrinkle free. Helps to protect the natural acid in the scalp and skin.
Cucumber (Khira)	Have natural astringent and cooling properties. Used for toning, refreshing, cooling and opening skin pores.
Genda (Marigold)	A flowering plant with several medicinal uses. Cures eczema and ringworm, used as a cleansing and healing lotion.
Honey (Shahad)	Used in many beauty treatments. Excellent for smoothing the skin and softens lines and wrinkles. Helps curing paralysis.
Haldi (Turmeric)	Besides used as spices in cooking, it helps prevent flatulence, cures injuries and wounds, poultices for boils, prevents inflammation, used for treating gonorrhea
Khus-khus (Poppy seed)	Cures insomnite, dry itch when rubbed with lime juice.

(Contd.

Name of Product	*Used Extensively for*
Lemon (Nimbu)	Have a bleaching, astringent action. Can be too drying for sensitive, parched skins but very good for oily, blemished ones. Brightens hair when used rinsing of hair after shampooing.
Milk	A vital source of calcium and vitamins. Regular drinking of milk ensures better nails, hair, teeth and skin complexion.
Oatmeal	Used as face pack for blackheads. If the skin is dry, mix with honey and apply face mask.
Olive oil (Jaitun tel)	Good for face, hair, nails and body for combating dryness.
Pudina (Mint)	Good for stomach ailments because of its digestive properties. Cures elephantiasis and varicose veins. Beneficial in case of curing urticaria.
Yoghurt (Dahi)	Has many beauty uses. Used as face mask. Good for unmanageable hair. Has cooling, softening, whitening and refreshing properties.

Constipation: May be defined as infrequent bowel evacuation or decreased frequency of usual bowel movements. If the stool are unusually hard, dry and difficult to expel, the patient is said to be constipated. The main causes include

1. **Habitual:** Addiction to tea, coffee and smoking, excessive use of laxatives and purgatives, old age (due to sluggish peristalsis), Pscyhogenic—change of place of evacuation, lack of exercise, errectic diet, insufficient food and water intake, use of drugs (belladonna/dhatura, narcotics, diuretics, salts of bismuth, calcium, iron, ammonium hydroxide and aluminum phosphatogel).
2. **Due to Certain Diseases:** Such as obstructive colonic disorders (Carcinoma of rectum, colon, T.B. of ileocaecal and congenital megacolon), absence of autonomic nerve plexus in a segment of colon, intestinal obstruction (due to round worms in children, T.B. of abdomen, weakness of intestinal system and abdominal muscles.

Signs and Symptoms: Which include cracked tongue, loss of appetite, headache and discomfort, pain in abdomen, flatulence in abdomen and other complications e.g. piles and ulcer. The following treatment is suggested:

(a) **Diet Therapy:** Adequate food intake, consumption of food having high fibre content (such as bran, raw fruits and vegetables) and adequate fluids (drinking at least eight glasses of water a day).

(b) **Yoga or Exercises:** To tone the external abdominal muscles *Ardha Matsyendra Asana, Ardha Vakra Asana, Dhanur Asana, Mayur Asana, Pawan-Mukta Asana, Uttan Pada Asana are recommended exercises* to relieve constipation and improve digestive system. Hip bath should be given regularly and abdominal massage followed by fomentation should be administered.

Fasting: It is used to cleanse the body of all the imbedded waste matter, remove the deep rooted toxins and give rest to the different organs of the body. In order to prepare the body for fasting begin with eating only raw vegetables for 4-5 days. For the next four days take only liquid diet including the juice of raw vegetables or fruits. Do not consume more than 4-5 glasses of liquid a day. Now, you are ready for complete fasting. Take only fresh lime with honey or plain water for next four to seven days. Just like you cannot begin fasting suddenly you cannot end it suddenly. The next four days take only raw or boiled vegetables. And slowly, over a period of ten days, you can come back to your original cereal diet. Many of the ailments e.g. acne, rheumatism, asthma, ulcers, alcoholism, heart disease and many other diseases just seem to dissolve while fasting.

Indigestion: Pain in the stomach, heart burn, tenderness over the stomach, badly coated tongue, acidity or belching of gas, headache, vomiting and pain in the back are common symptoms of chronic indigestion. These are caused due to eating too fast, partially cooked foods habit, use of intoxicant liquors, indulging in desk work, untimely meals, eating between meals, late hour eating, emotional upsets, severe mental strain and constipation generally cause indigestion. The treatment include eating well balanced, well cooked, well chewed food. Do not over eat. Eat only when you are hungry. Never eat when you are tired, emotionally upset and anxious. Enema should be given at the time of commencement of the treatment to clean bowels. Hot fomentation, mud pack on abdomen daily and cold hip bath twice a day, oil massage and mud bath are beneficial in curing indigestion and dyspepsia. Avoid taking seets, fried food, spiced foods, processed foods and sour things.

Surya Namaskar Asana: This asana involves various bending forward and backward postures and can prove to be excellent caretaker of the health if practiced regularly before doing yogic postures and pranayama. Stand straight keeping the legs apart 12 to 24 inches, with hands hanging loosely at sides. Look in front and breathe normally. Lower the upper area of the body bending forward towards the ground, exhaling (elbow or palms touching the floor) keeping legs and spine straight. Rest for 6 to 8 seconds and return to the standing position till you finish inhaling. Rest and repeat the exercise 3 to 4 times. This asana has several benefits i.e. activates all the glands of the endocrinal system (the pancreas, adrenal, thyroid, pituitary and some other glands begin to secrete their respective hormones). It leaves good effect on the stomach, spine, lungs and chest. The asana invigorates the facial tissues, the central nerve system and all the organs of the upper part of the body, Surya Namaskar Asana comprises of the following positions:

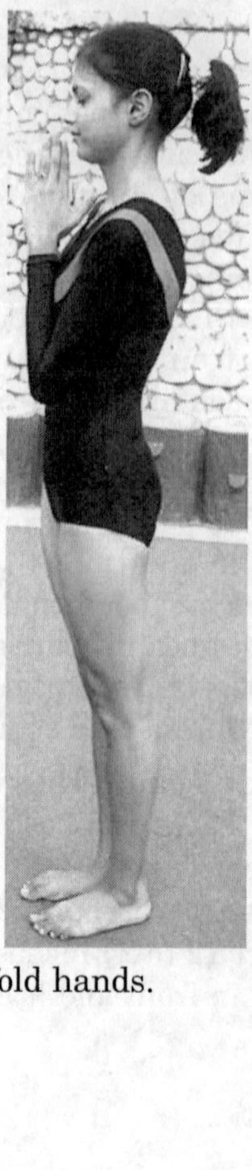

1. Stand erct and fold hands.

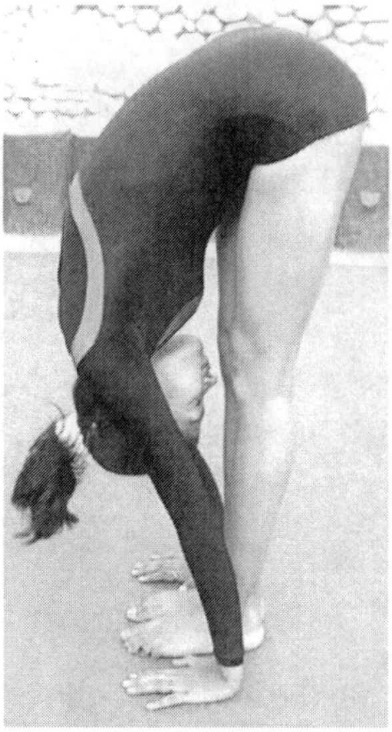

2. Inhale slowly and raise both arms upward, stretched. Bend downward, touching the floor with both hands.

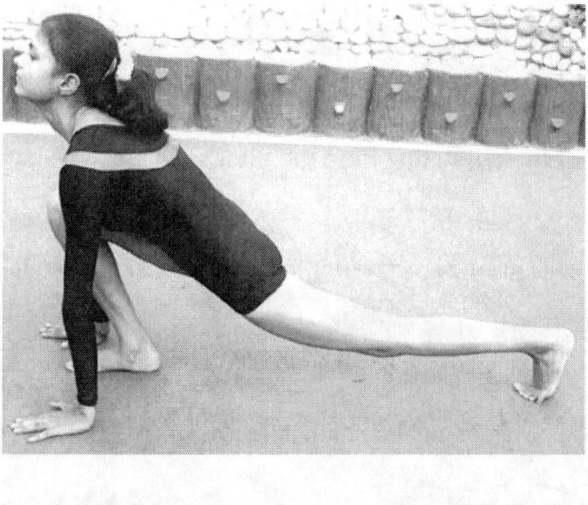

3. Hold breath for a few seconds, then put both the hands on the floor raising the head and stretching the left leg backward.

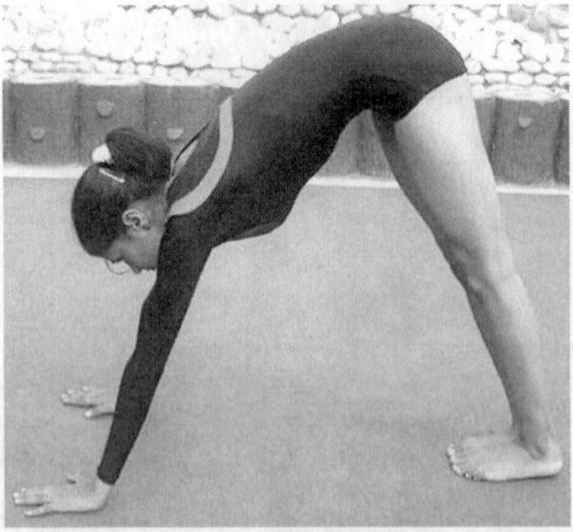

4. Stretch right leg too and raise the body.

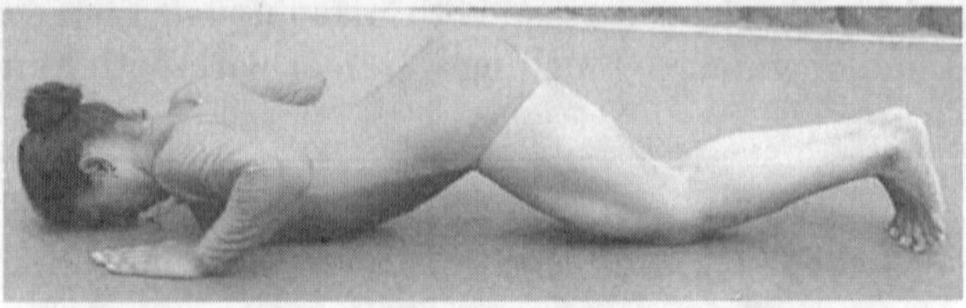

5. Lower the chest, touching the floor with chin.

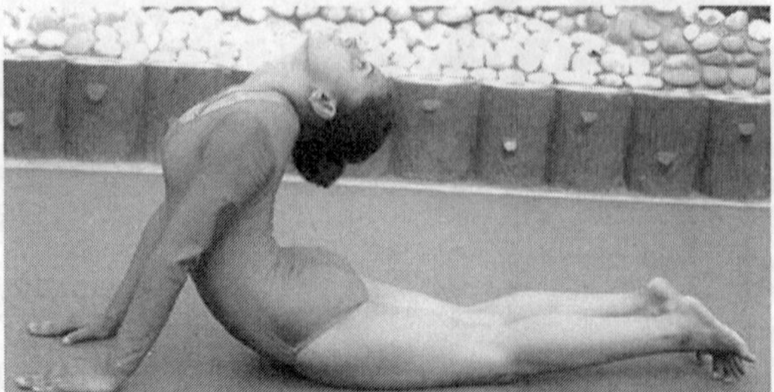

6. Raise head, trunk, hips, thighs and knees from floor.

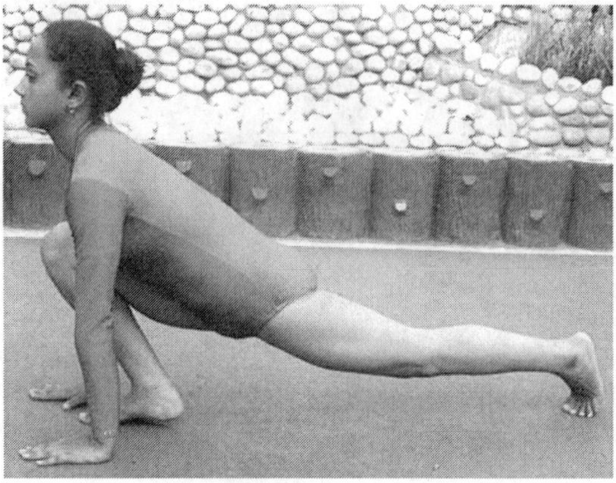

7. Bring right foot forward and left leg stretched back.

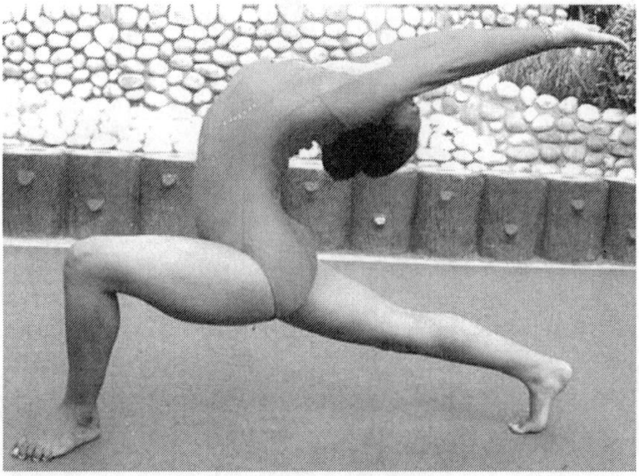

8. Raise the body with hands backward.

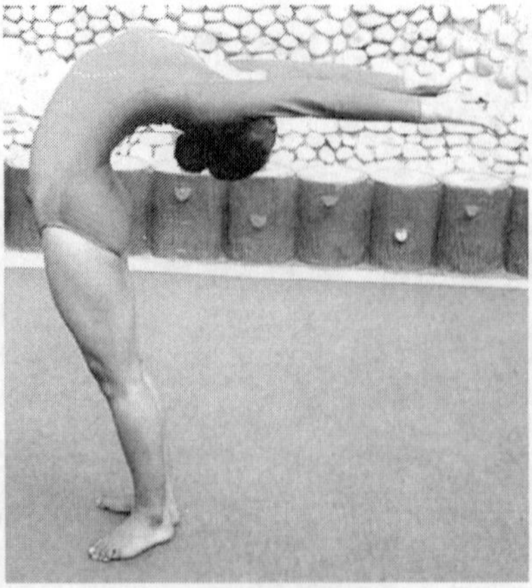

9. Bend backward with raised hands and feet joined.

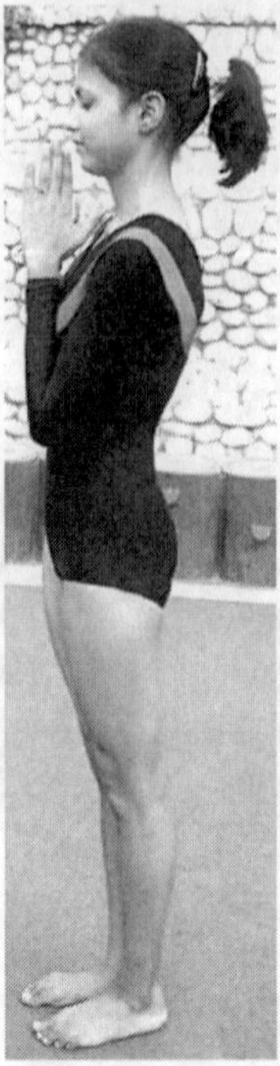

10. Return to the original standing position with folded hands.

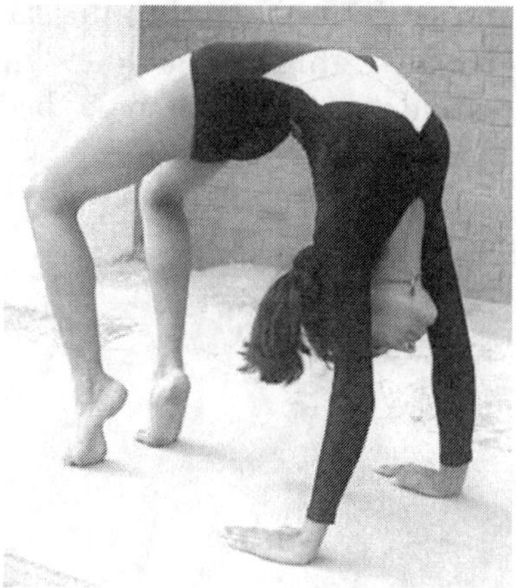

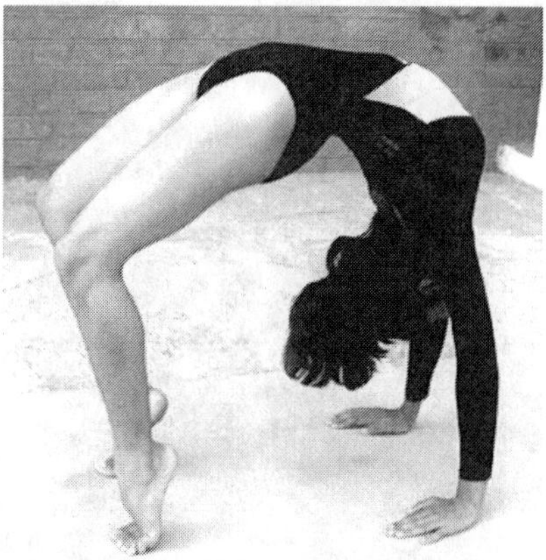

Chakara Asana (Wheel Posture): In this posture the body is made to appear like a wheel which is a good stretching exercise to almost all the skeletal muscles. To do this asana, lie on your back. Bring your palms under the shoulders. Now raise your back and buttocks off the floor. Curve your spine resting the crown of your head on the floor. Straighten your arms and arch your spine upwards as high as possible. This is Chakra Asana. The therapeutic advantages includes: it renders the spinal column flexible and strengthen the muscles of the abdomen, thighs, shoulders and arms. This asana regenerates kidneys, helps to make body strong and energetic.

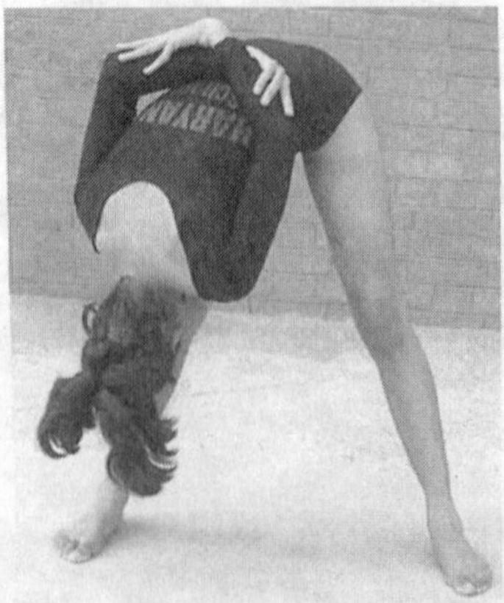

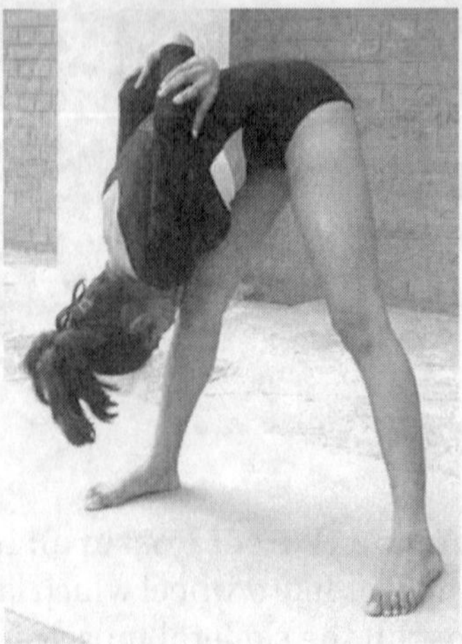

Kona Asana (Angel Posture): This posture renders the spinal column and hip joints supple. It tones up the abdominal organs and removes stiffness in the legs. In this asana stand erect with 18 to 24 inches distance apart in both feet. Lean forward touching head to the right knee and hands behind on the back. Remain in this position for 6-8 seconds. Repeat this asana 4 to 6 times on each side.

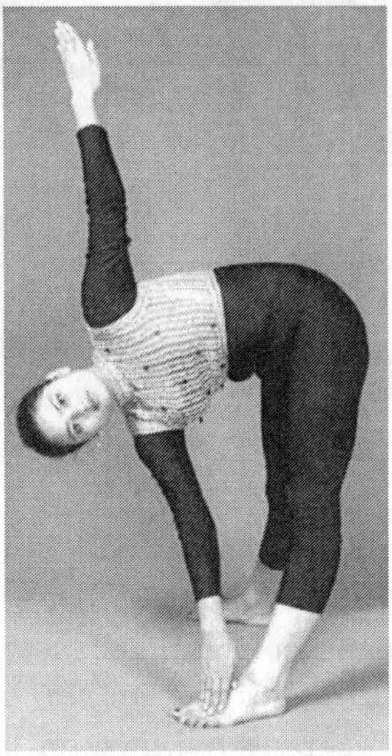

Trikona Asana (Triangle Posture): Stand with the legs apart. Rotate waist, begin to exhale until the fingers of the right hand touch the ground. Hold for some time, stand up, perform the same movement to the other hand. This posture makes the entire body strong and elastic. It tones up the muscles in the back, the hips and legs.

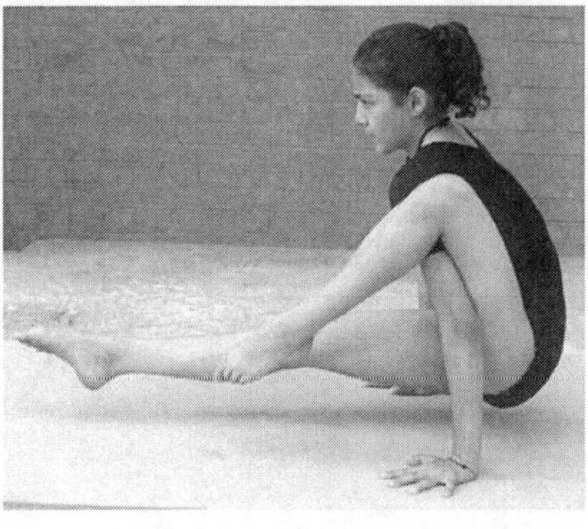

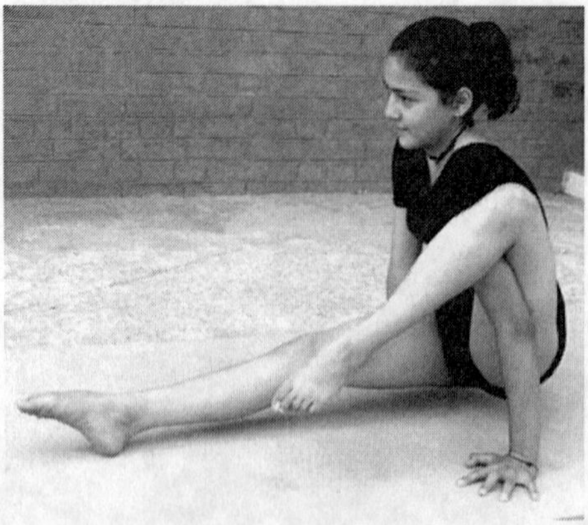

Ek Hasta Bhujang Asana: This is a posture of the leg supported by the arm. Sit on the floor which arms on the sides and palms resting on the floor. Keep right by straight on the floor and left leg resting on the left shoulder. Now raise hips upwards keeping balance on both arms. Stay in this position for 5 to 6 seconds and lower the body on the floor. Rest and repeat the asana 4 to 5 times. This posture strengthens the abdominal muscles, fortifies the arms, wrists and hands.

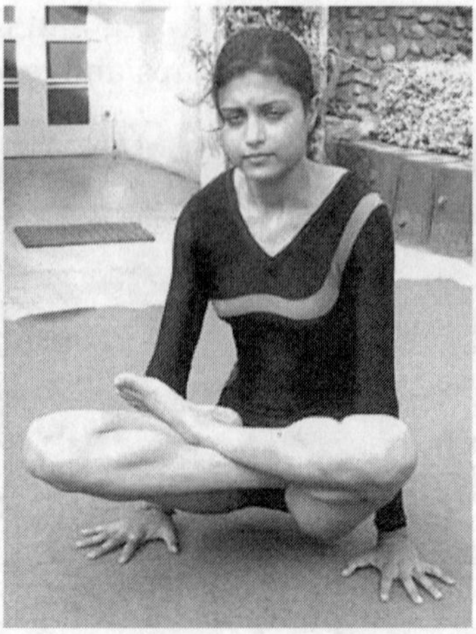

Kukkuta Asana: Kukkuta means a cock sit in Padmasana. Insert your arms into the gaps between the calves and thighs, palms touching the floor. Raise your thighs and hips off the floor. Balance the body. This asana strengthen the fingers, wrists, arms and abdomen muscles.

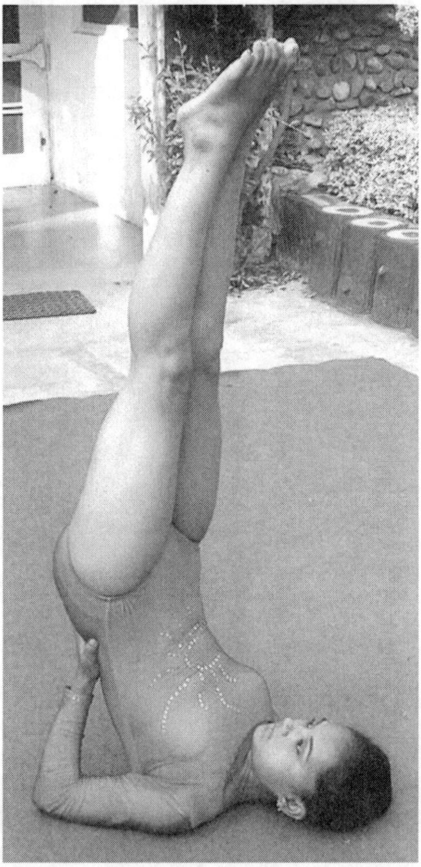

Sarvang Asana (Position 1)

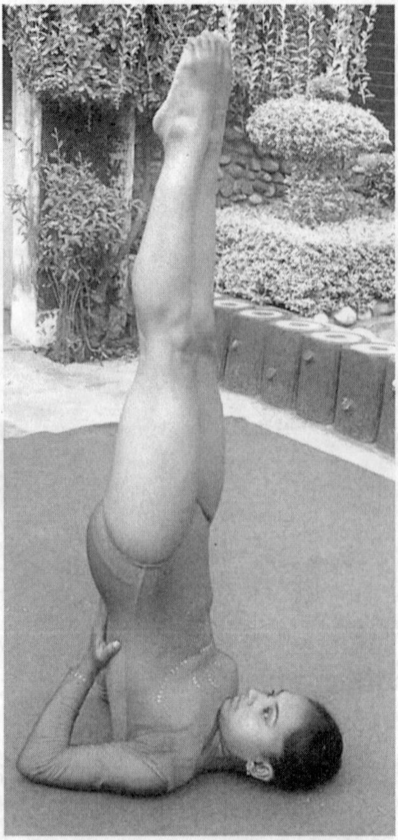

Sarvang Asana (Position 2)

Sarvang Asana: Sarva means all and anga means parts. Lie on your back, bend your knees towards the chest. Raise your hips and legs off the floor supporting back with your palms. Straighten your legs perpendicular to the floor. This asana helps relieve headaches, colds, cough, constipation and improves functioning of all organs, glands and nerves.

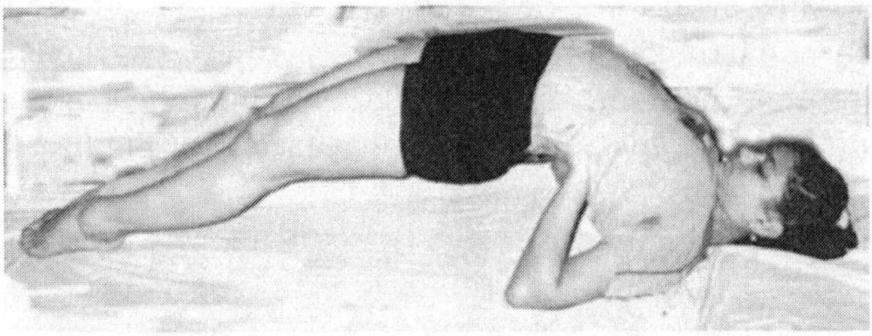

The therapeutic advantages of this posture are similar to Sarvanga Asana. It helps to fight overweight around hips thighs and waist.

Setubandha Sarvang Asana: Setu means bridge and bandha means construction. This pose is a variation of Sarvang-asana. Keep your buttocks raised and bend your knees backwards. Tighten your buttocks and arch your back. Return to Sarvang Asana and lie flat on your back. This asana strengthens the wrist, tones up the kidney, makes spine strong, improves breathing, refreshes the body and mind.

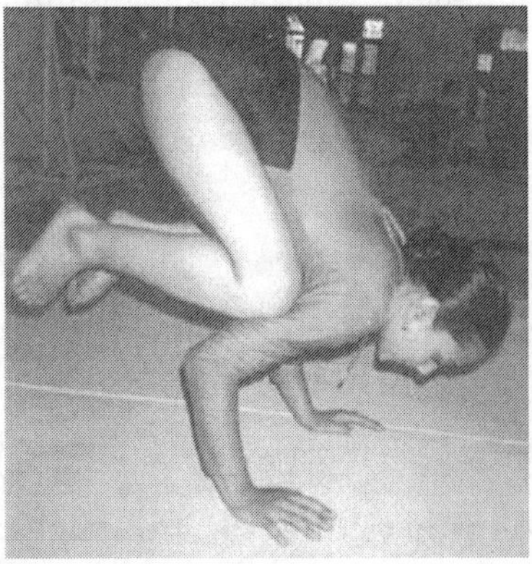

Bak Asana (Crow Posture): Baka means a crane squat, spread knees placing palms on the floor near the feet.

Raise hips and the head resting your knees on the upper arms. Now sway your body forward. Raise foot off the floor one by one balancing the arms. This asana strengthens arm wrists and shoulder, muscles. This challenging pose gives strength, confidence and improves concentration.

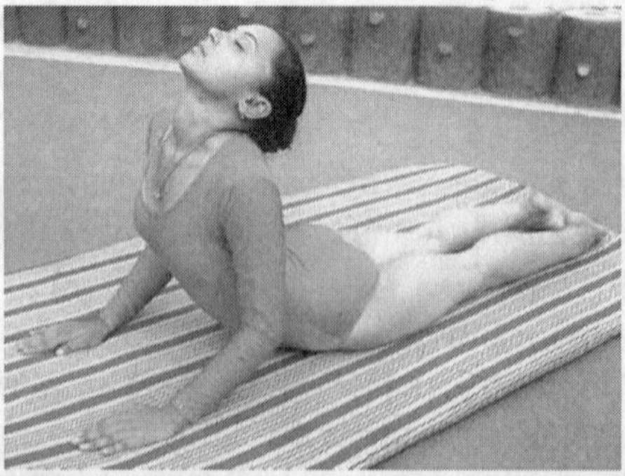

Ardha Bhujang Asana (Easy Cobra Position): It is an easy yoga posture of Bhujang Asana, lie on your stomach. Raise your trank off the floor and throw your headback. This asana helps to tone up spinal column, activates abdominal area, leaves beneficial effect on adrenal glands, stimulates digestion and soothes backaches.

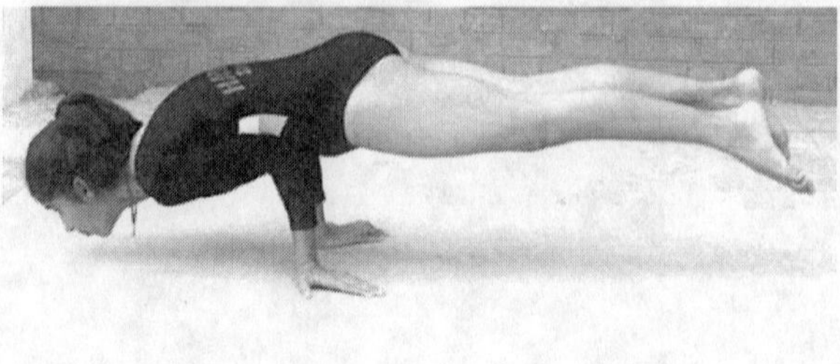

Mayur Asana (Peacock Posture): Kneel on the ground, knees apart, palms flat on the floor, fingers pointing towards the fact, brining the elbows under the abdomen just under the navel. Lean forward to touch the ground with forehead and stretching out the leg behind raising the feet and head and keep body horizontal (parallel to the ground). Stay balanced on the arms as long as possible, then lie down on the stomach. This posture increases supply of blood to the digestive organs and cures constipation. It tones up the abdomal muscles and brings the body into equilibrium. This asana fortifies, the hand, wrist and forearms.

5

Yoga Exercises for Facial and Body Beauty

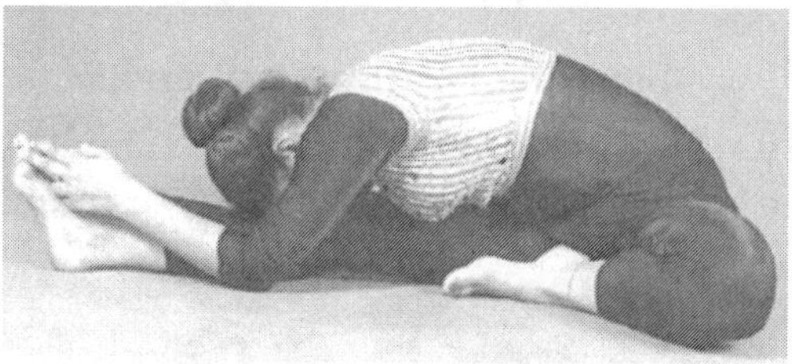

Janusir Asana: This asana as shown in the illstration which helps to strengthen the muscles of spinal column, supple the muscles of legs and back. The asana is especially good for the menstruation disorders. The standing posture of Janusira Asana is known as Dandya-mana Janusir Asana which has the similar therapeutic advantages.

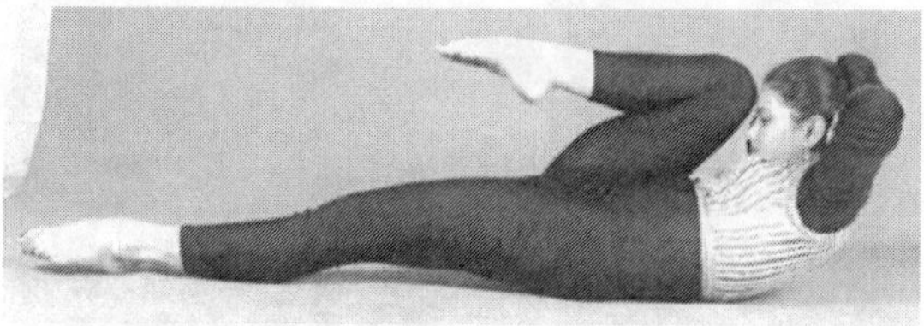

Janusir Merudanda Asana (Position 1)

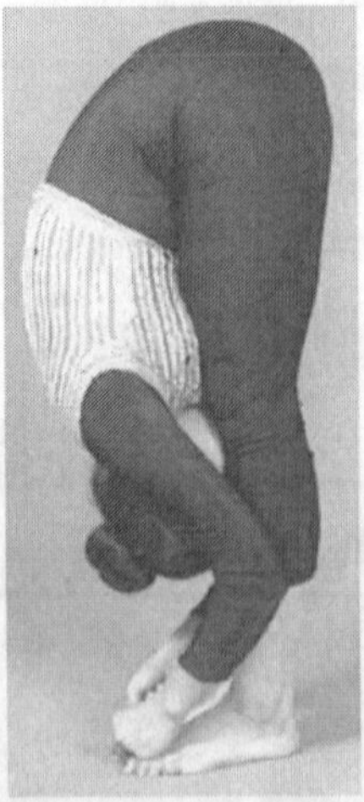

Standing Posture (Position 2)

Janusir Merudanda Asana: The therapeutic advantage of this yogic posture is similar to Janusira Asana.

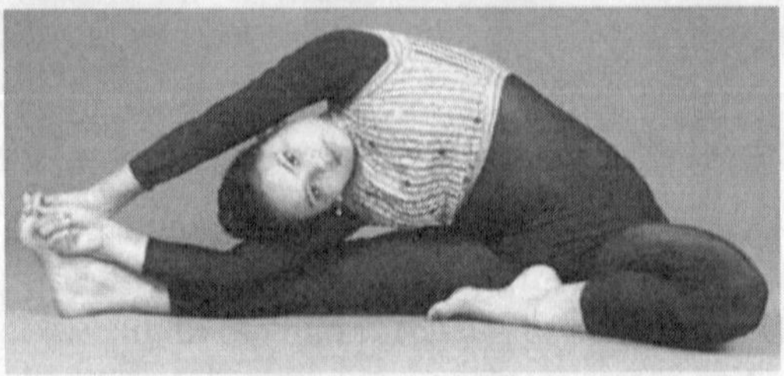

Parivritta Janusir Asana: The therapeutic advantage of this exercise is similar to Janusir Asana.

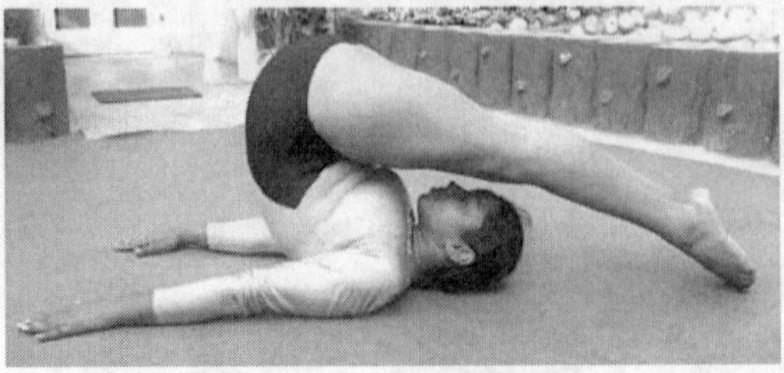

Hal Asana (Position 1)

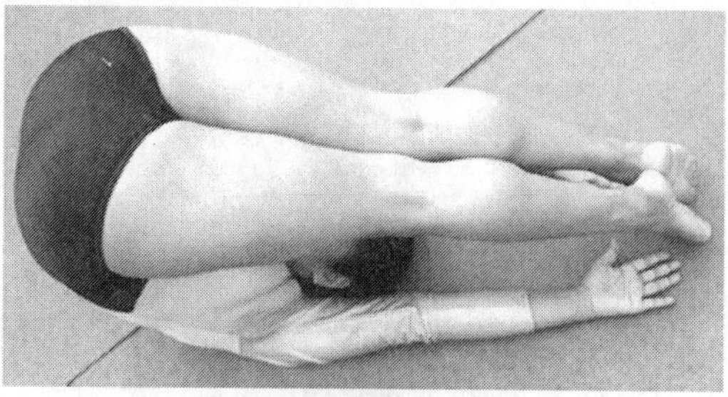

(Position 2)

Hal Asana (Plough Posture): Lie on the back, arms stretched by the side. Raise the legs slowly stretched vertically. Then lower the legs behind the head until the tips of the feet touch the ground. Remain in this position for 20-40 seconds breathing regularly. Return to the starting position. Relax and repeat the posture. Do not strain if you have a stiff spinal column. Hala Asana keeps the spinal supple and healthy, helps relieve digestive problems, increases supply of blood, revitalizes the nerves and muscles of back and have regenerating effect on the glandular system, clears menstrual disorders, prevents fat from forming on stomach, waist and hips and removes exhaustion and fatigue.

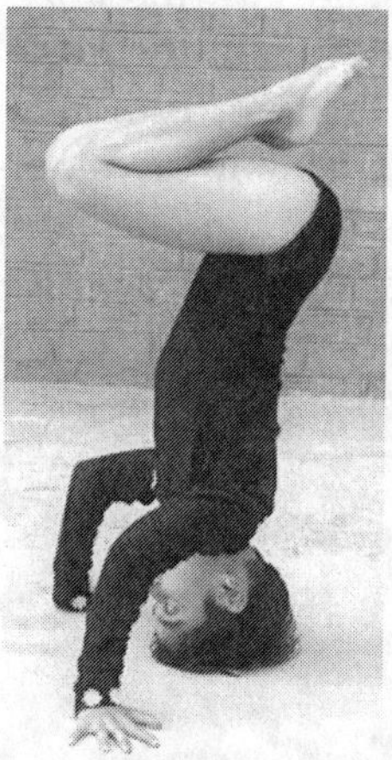

Sirsh Asana (Initial Position)

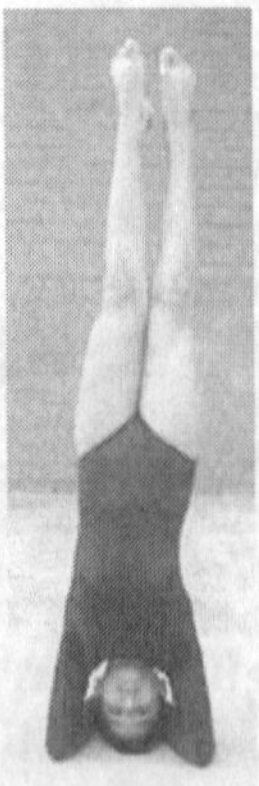

Sirsh Asana (Final Position)

Sirsh Asana (Head Stand posture): This yogic asana is also called "The king of Asanas". Kneel in front resting forearms, interlocked fingers on head. Slowly raise the knees and the hips, knees off the ground in steps. Straighten legs perpendicular to the floor. Remain in this position for some time, then return to initial position. If you are unable to practice this asana, learn the posture taking support of the wall. Lift shoulders. Throw your legs backward or forward slowly. Therapeutic advantages of this asana include increased blood circulation in the head and upper portion of the body, removes fatigue, builds up energy, improves concentration and will power, strengthen entire body, promote growth, have beneficial effect on endocrine and digestive system and increase facial beauty.

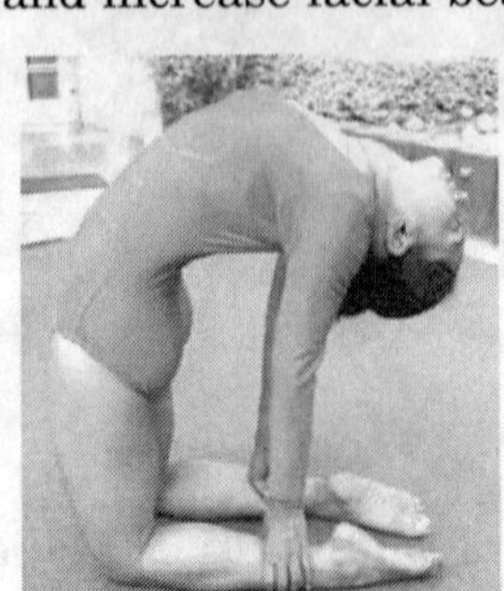

Ushtra Asana (Camel Posture): This asana helps remove stiffness in the neck and shoulders, cures visionary and voice defects, throat troubles, tonsils, chronic headache and respiratory system. The asana activates the facial tissues and strengthens the muscles of

Kneel with your toes pointing backwards, rest your hands on hips, curve back. Drop your palms one by one on to the soles of your feet. This is Ushtra-asana. Stay in this position for 6 to 8 seconds, then come up. Repeat the exercise three to four times.

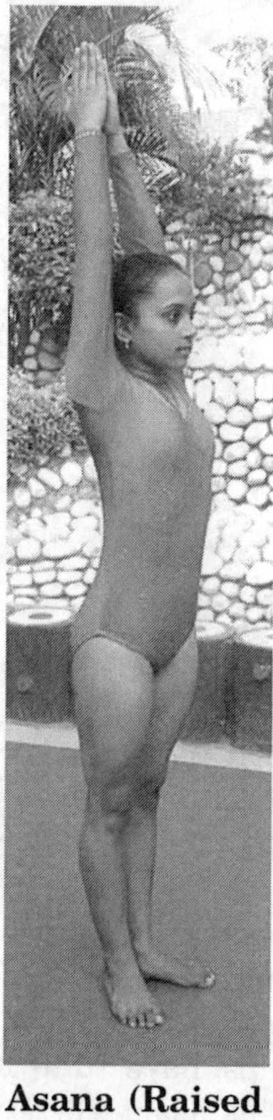

Urdhva Hasta Asana (Raised Arm Posture): This exercise is beneficial for correct standing posture especially

for children. It makes the back straight, strong and the mind alert. Stand straight with equal weight on both feet. Avoid protrude your buttocks and hold breath when stretching your arms overhead.

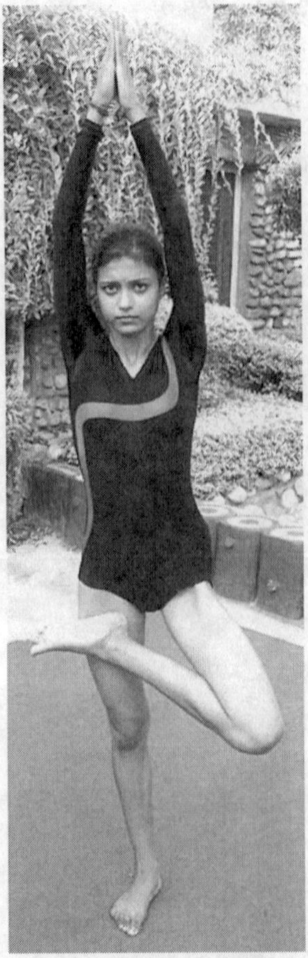

Vriksha Asana: Have many benefits e.g. health, strength, flexibility, concentration and grace. Stand straight. Stretch arms up and place right foot on left upper thigh. Rest hands on your hips, have 10 to 15 counts. Repeat the pose on other side. This asana corrects posture, improves concentration and balance, strengthens legs, arms and shoulders.

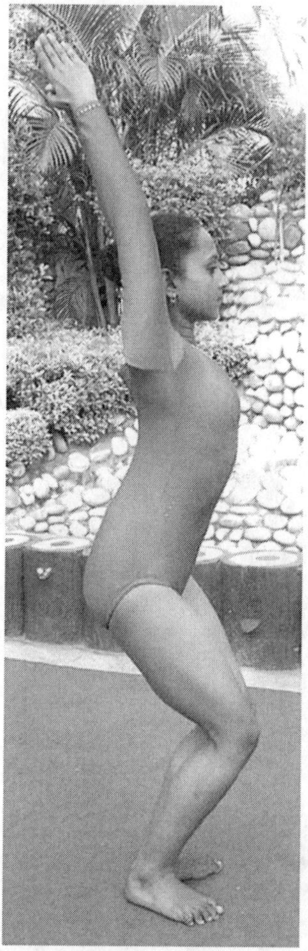

Utkata Asana (High, Mighty or Superior): Stand straight. Stretch your arms upwards joining palms. Look straight ahead, and bend your knees imaging you are sitting on a chair. Have count 5 to 10 times. This exercise strengthens the ankles, calves, arms, legs, ankles, inner thighs and back.

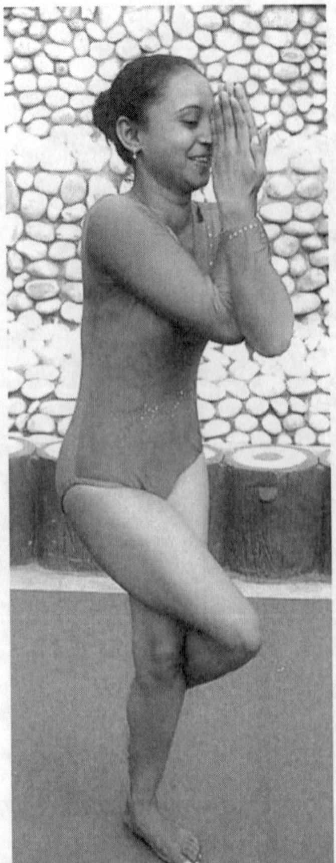

Garuda Asana: Garuda with the body of a man and the head, wings and claws of an eagle. An asana to strengthen the whole body. It relieves cramps in the calves. Stand straight looking ahead. Bend knees placing your left leg over around the right and simultaneously place your one arm over and around the other. Repeat the pose on the other leg having 10 to 12 counts on each side.

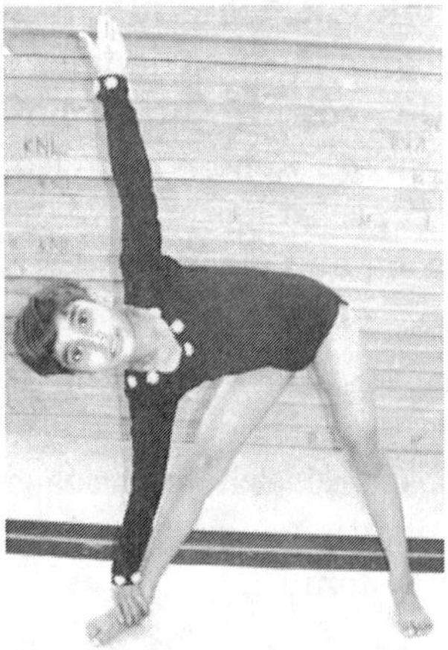

Utthita Trikona Asana: Utthita means extended, Tri means three and kona means angle—thus Trikona means triangle. This pose helps strengthening the whole body, especially beneficial for building up the chest, improving the arches of the feet, shaping the legs and the ankles. To do this posture, jump and spread your legs 2 to 3 feet apart with arms side ways. Now bend on a side touching palms on the ankle or floor. Stretch opposite arm up and look up at the fingertips. Return to standing position and repeat the pose on other side. Make 10 to 15 counts each side.

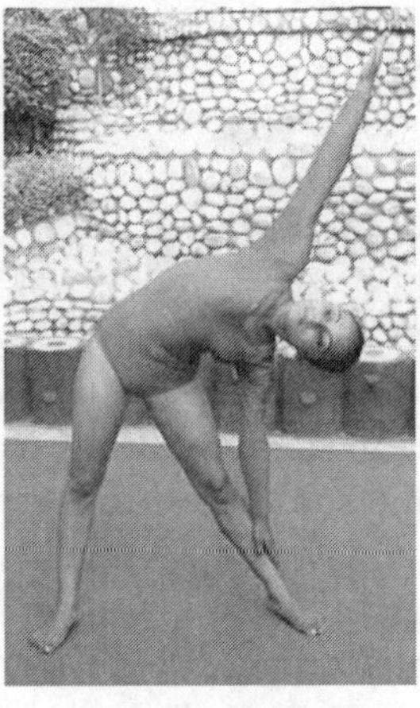

Parivritta Trikona Asana: Parivritta means twisted or revolved and trikona means triangle. This is the twisted triangle pose. In this posture, turn your right foot out 90° and your left foot in 45°. Repeat exercise on other side. Do not let your thigh muscles loosen. This posture, too makes the entire body strong and elastic and strengthen the back. Have 10 to 15 counts each side.

Vira Bhadra Asana (Warrior Pose): This yogic posture comprises of three poses as shown in the photographs. These exercises help increase stamina, improve balance and concentration, strengthen muscles of the chest, shoulders, back and stomach.

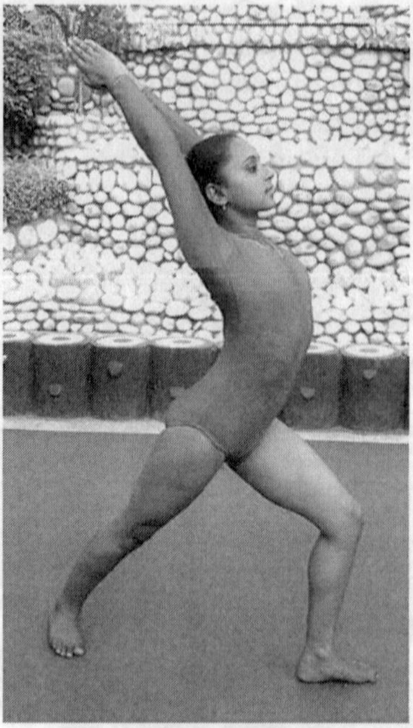

Posture 1: Stand straight. Jump and spread legs 3 to 4 feet apart with arms side ways. Raise your arms up. Turn right foot out 90° and left in 45°. Revolve your hips and turn your trunk to the right. Look up at your fingertips. Return to initial position and repeat the pose on left side.

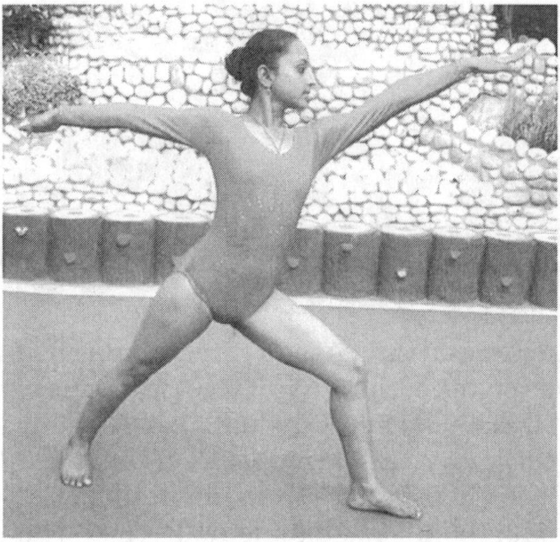

Posture 2: Bend your right knee to form a right angle and look at your right fingertips.

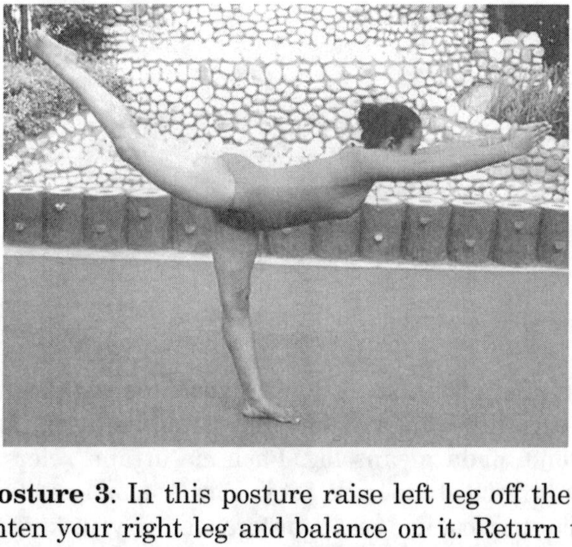

Posture 3: In this posture raise left leg off the floor, straighten your right leg and balance on it. Return to the original position and repeat the pose on the left side. This asana builds stamina and improves balance and concentration.

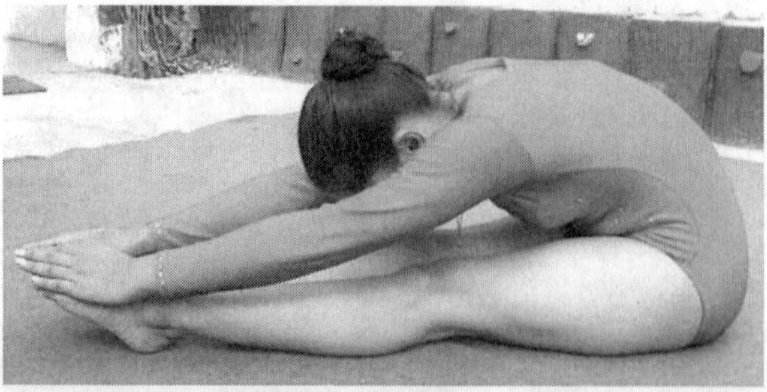

Paschima-uttana Asana (Stretching the Back and Legs): Lie on the back with feet together. Raise arms above the head inhaling. Sit up, exhaling. Lean forward until head touches the knees. Hold big toe of feets with the thumb and index finger of hands and stay in this position for 7 seconds, then gradually sit up. Exhale and relax. This posture strengthens the organs of the abdomen and spinal column, regenerates kidneys and digestive organs, relieves constipation, cures diabetes and prevents formation of fat around stomach and back.

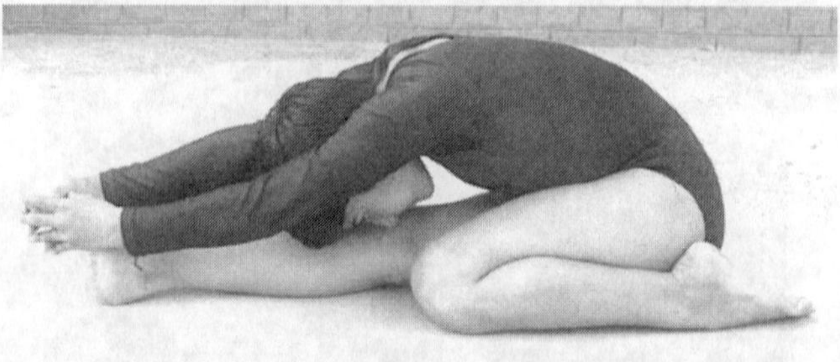

Tri-anga Mukha-ek-pada Paschima-uttana-Asana: Tri means three, anga means limbs, mukha means face, ek mean one, pada means leg. Pachima-uttana refers to an intense stretch of the back. Sit in Vira Asana, bend forward, hold your left foot and rest your forehead on your knee. Avoid tilting your body to a side. This asana strengthens and shapes the muscles of legs, hips, spine and abdomen organs.

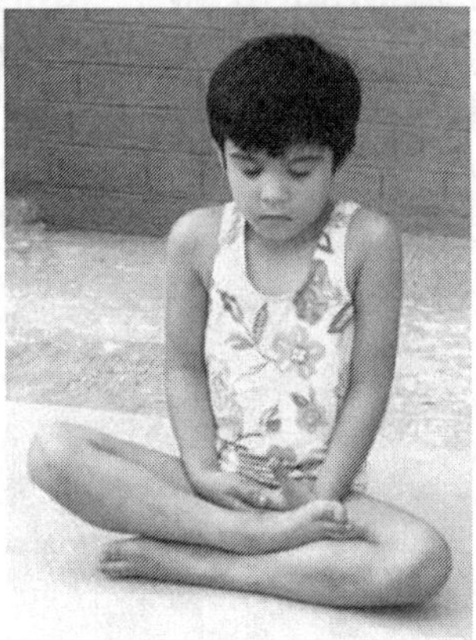

Ardha Baddha Padma Paschima Uttana Asana (Strecthing the Back and Hips): Sit in Padma asana. Raise arms up inhaling, lean forwarding exhaling, bend forward until head touches the knee. Practice this asana not more than 3 times in a day. This asana makes back supple, regenerates the kidneys, good remedy for constipation, prevents the formulation of fat around back, abdomen, stomach and waist. It stimulates glands of prostate, uterus and bladder.

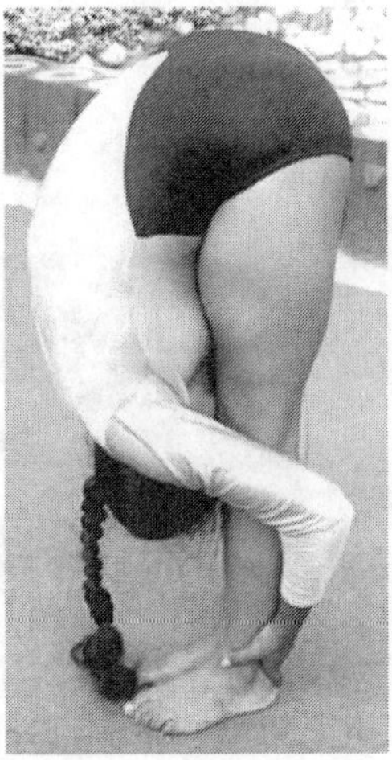

Ourdhva Paschimottan Asana: Ourdhva means upward. The asana stretches the back and legs upward. The therapeutic advantages of this asana are similar to those of Paschimottan Asana. The posture exercise, develop equilibrium, mental stability and power of concentration.

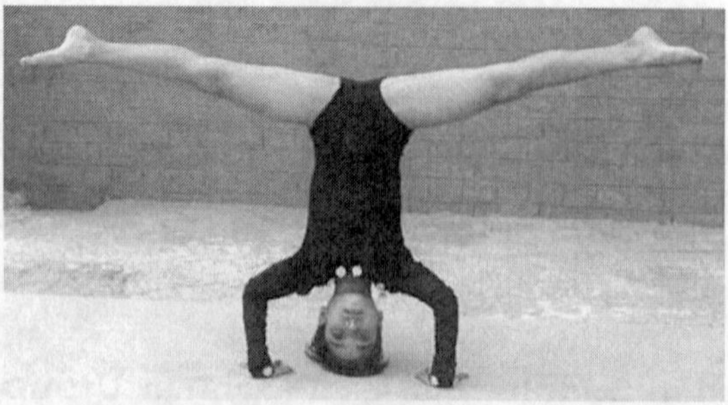

Salambha Sirsh Asana: The therapeutic advantages of this yoga exercise are similar to those of Sirsha Asana. The body is held straight, up-side down, on the head. It promotes circulation and removes congestion of blood. To do this, take position of Sirsha Asana and bring both legs horizontal parallel to the ground. This posture is extremely beneficial for the facial skin, scalp disorders, hair loss and disorders of gentio urinary and reproductive organs.

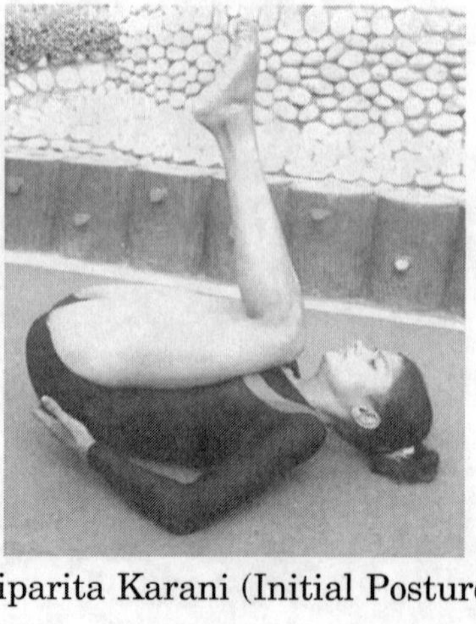

Viparita Karani (Initial Posture)

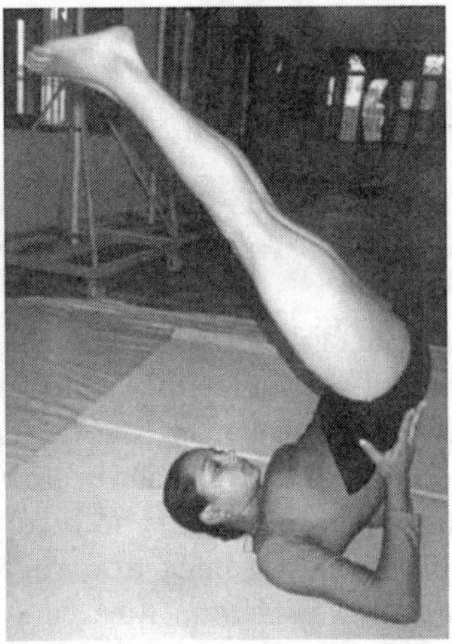

Viparita Karani (Final Posture)

Viparitakarani (Inverted Posture): In Sanskirt Viparita means inverted and karani means action. Lie on the back and inhale. Raise legs and hips with the help of arms and exhale. The legs should form and angle of 60° to 70°. Lower the legs gently to the ground and relax. Repeat the exercise two to three times. If you suffer from high blood pressure, patients are suggested to consult a doctor before doing exercise. This posture is beneficial for reviving the body, prevents formation of facial wrinkels, regenerates thyroid and pituitary glands, nervous system, posture and flow of blood to the neck, throat and head.

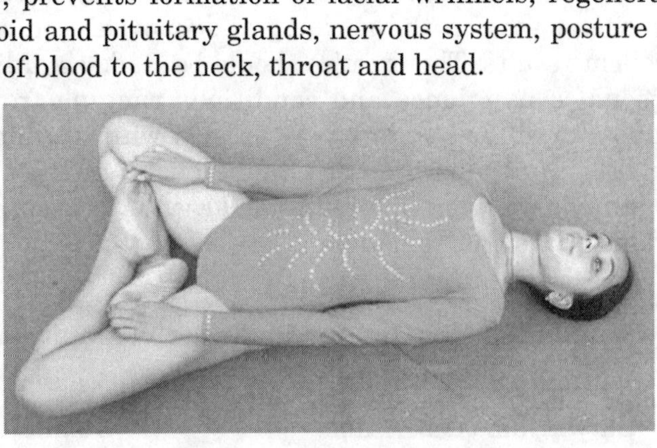

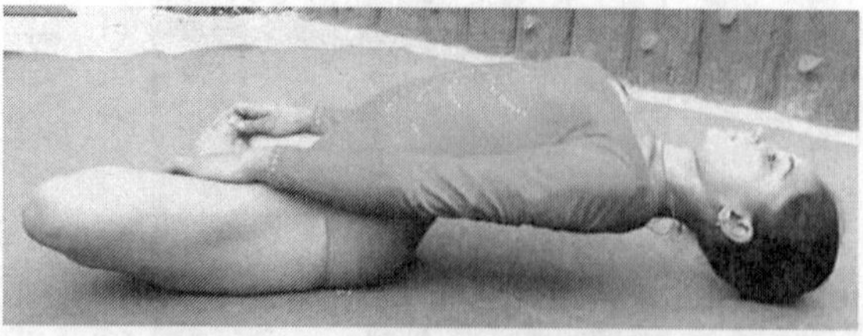

Matsya Asana (Fish Posture): Sit in Padmasana. Inhale, then exhale. Lean the trunk backwards with the help of elbows. Lift the chest upwards, rest the crown of the head on the floor. Take hold of the big toes breathing lightly. Hold the posture for one to 2 minutes, then return to the starting position, relax lying on the back and repeat asana 3 to 4 times. This asana strengthens and regenerates thyroid glands, leaves beneficial effect on the spinal column, renders the neck supple, removes all aches and stiffness, stretch neck muscles, provoke on abundant flow of blood to entire body, fortifies back muscles, keeps abdominal organs healthy and refresh the body and mind.

Thirty Minutes Daily Yoga Routine to Keep Fit

The regular practice of yoga asanas in tables below will be beneficial to maintain good health and prevent recurrence of body disorders the practitioner suffer from. A sound mental is a key to good health and beauty of your body. A regular practice of yoga in the morning and/or evening provides excellent results. The practice should be made according to personal convenience and conditions ranging from 15 minutes to an hour. Start yoga session with warming up exercises. You must practice Shave Asana at the end of programme even for 15 minutes, followed by concentration and meditation for sometime.

Table I

Recommended Routine for Beginners (30 minutes)

Warming up exercises:	5 minutes
Surya Namaskar Asana:	5 minutes

Padma Asana:	2 minutes
Gomukh Asana:	2 minutes
Tara Asana:	3 minutes
Pawan Mukta Asana:	1 minute
Bhujang Asana:	1 minute
Trikona Asana:	2 minutes
Shallabh Asana:	1 minute
Ek Pada Uttan/Uttanpada Asana:	2 minutes
Yog Mudra:	1 minute
Shava Asana:	5 minutes

Table II

Recommended Routine for Children (15 minutes)

Warming up exercises:	3 minutes
Surya Namaskar Asana:	3 minutes
Urdhava Hasta Asana:	30 seconds
Vriksha Asana:	30 seconds
Utkata Asana:	30 seconds
Ardh Chandera Asana:	30 seconds
Vir Bhadra Asana (3-Postures):	2 minutes
Simha Asana:	30 seconds
Adho Mukha Shvana Asana:	30 seconds
Paschimottan Asana:	1 minute
Yog Mudra Asana:	30 seconds
Shava Asana:	3 minutes

Table III

Recommended Postures for Women (30 minutes)

Warming up exercises:	3 minutes
Surya Namaskar Asana:	4 minutes

Padma Asana:	1 minute
Gomukh Asana:	1 minute
Bhujang Asana/Dhanur Asana:	1 minute
Ushtra Asana:	1 minute
Paśchimoottan Asana:	1 minute
Sarvang Asana:	1 minute
Supt-Vajra Asana:	1 minute
Ek-Pada Uttan Asana:	1 minute
Pawan Mukta Asana:	1 minute
Janusir Asana:	1 minute
Shallabh Asana:	1 minute
Yog Mudra/Viparitakarani:	2 minutes
Manduk Asana:	2 minutes
Simha Asana:	1 minute
Vajroli Mudra:	1 minute
Ardh Vakra/Ardh Matsyendra Asana:	1 minute
Shav Asana:	5 minutes

Table IV

Recommended Postures for Pregnants (15 minutes)

Light Warming up Exercises:	2 minutes
Meditation:	3 minutes
Yog Mudra:	1 minute
Pawan Mukta Asana (lying on back):	1 minute
Ardh Bhujang Asana:	1 minute
Tara Asana:	1 minute
Marjara Asana:	1 minute
Shav Asana:	5 minutes

Table V

Recommended Postures for Adults (30 Minutes)

Warming up exercise:	4 minutes
Meditation:	2 minutes
Padmasana:	2 minutes
Yog Mudra:	2 minutes
Bhujang Asana:	2 minutes
Dhanur Asana/Chakra Asana:	2 minutes
Ushtra-Asana/Viprita Karni:	2 minutes
Sarvang Asana:	2 minutes
Hal Asana:	2 minute
Matsyendra Asana/Vakra Asana:	1 minute
Shallabh Asana:	1 minute
Sirsh Asana/Salamba Sirsh Asana:	2 minutes
Shav Asana:	5 minutes

(The duration of this routine can be increased to 60 minutes after sufficient practice)

6

Yogic Cure for Genito-Urinary Disorders and Reproductive System

Faulty Functioning of Ovaries: Symptoms include *Amenorrhoea* (absence of menstrual flow in women), *Menorrhagia* (Excessive bleeding during menstruation) and Metrorrahagia (excessive bleeding from the uterus from onset of the puberty or any age. Recommended yogic exercises: *Paranayama, Dhanur Asana, Halasana, Mal Asana, Sarvang Asana, Sirsh Asana.*

Female Diseases: Symptoms include *Leucorrhoea* (vaginal discharge may be associated with a viscid, thick, foul smell generally due indigestion and sedentary habit).

Displacement of Uterus or uterine prolapse (usually occurs after delivery or in women who are aged and given birth to too many children. The uterus slips downwards in between the space of the bladder and bowel. It may produce from the vagina with offensive smell sometimes due to infection. Recommended yogic exercises: *Gomukh Asana, Manduk Asana, Yog Mudra, Upavista, Kona Asana, Shallabh Asana, Pachimottan Asana, Matsya Asana.*

Vaginitis (Blood stained discharge): Due to infection or erosion of the cervix. It is an alarming sign of problem pregnancy. Consult a doctor for suitable yoga exercises.

White Vaginal Discharge: Usually due to local infection of vagina or cervix with symptoms of severe itching, burning and sometimes heavy yellowish flow. Recommended postures: *Matsaya Asana, Shallabh Asana, Ek Pada Uttan Asana.*

Pregnancy Toxemia: Causes abrupt occurrence of bleeding. The symptoms include sudden increase in weight, swelling in the body, rise in blood pressure, appearance of albumin in urine, breathlessness, diuretics to flush out urine. Very light yogic exercises are recommended.

Breast Inflammation: Causes in pregnant women. The main symptoms are belching, soreness in throat and loss of taste. Recommended postures *Bhujang Asana, Chakra Asana, Dhanur Asana.*

Stomach or Liver Pain: Due to increased weight of the embryo which results stained nerves. Massage stomach slowly with ghee to relieve pain. *Pranayama* is recommended.

Morning Sickness: Causes vomiting sensation during early stage of pregnancy or after two week beyond the scheduled date of regular menses. Recommended postures: *Marjara Asana, Tara Asana, Vira Asana, Uttana Asana.*

Dark Spots and Pigmented Lines on the Skin: The texture of the skin is affected during pregnancy which becomes fairer or darker due to action of sex hormones. The patches of dark spots usually appear on the face and various parts of the body including neck, back, abdomen and upper thighs due to stretching of the skin. Recommended posture: *Janusir Asana, Janusir Merudanda Asana, Parivrtta Asana.*

Tumour or Sores in the Uterus: Pain due to lesions in the uterus are caused. A vaginal douche with water in which neem leaves have been boiled relieves pain. Fermentation of the lower abdomen and the pubes by a cloth pad soaked in this decoction cures. The patient should eat easily digestible food. Avoid sex during this period.

Recommended postures: *Matsya Asana, Supta Vajra Asana, Hal Asana, Ardh Sarvanga Asana.*

Dysmenorrhoea: A sense of weakness and pain (in the groin also) proceeds the menstrual flow is a sign of irritation in the ovaries usually caused by inflammation of internal organs like womb, the ovaries or the fallopian tubes. Recommended prostures: *Tikona Asana, Vajroli Mudra, Ushtra Asana, Mal Asana, Gomukh Asana.*

Metritis: An inflammation of the uterus due to malfunctioning of the ovaries in which exercises similar to Dysmenorrhoea are recommended.

Flaccidity of the Breasts: The mammary glands of the breasts of women undergo many changes when lactation has begun. The breasts become firm and beautiful when a woman is suckling her infant. The firmness is reduced when lactation has stopped or a woman has gone beyond the childbearing age. The breast has a tendency to sag and become flaccid. Apply a paste of roots of the Banyan tree ground with water on the breast for a week. Recommended postures: *Bhujang Asana, Dhanur Asana.*

Premature Separation of Placenta: It is a worst disease may cause during advanced stage of pregnancy when the vaginal orifice starts widening or at the time of actual delivery approaches. The portion of the placenta which has already coagulated near vaginal orifice gets burst and is immediately followed by Haemorrhagia. An immediate medical treatment is essential to avoid trouble. Regular practice of few light exercises such as *Padma Asana, Baddha Kona Asana* (as advised by Naturopath) during the pregnancy period strengthen reproductive organs.

Cramps: The trouble in pregnants starts in the fourth month from conception when the pain shoots-up in the night while lying down to sleep. Cramping trouble develops due to deficiency of minerals and vitamins in the body. The pain develops more in waist, stomach, buttock muscles. Massage whole body with 'Narayana Oil'. Recommended postures: *Pas*

Asana, Manduk Asana, Garuda Asana, Parasarita Pada Uttan Asana, Gomukh Asana.

Delayed Menstruation: The trouble is seen in teenagers. Sometimes, the gap between the period is as longer two month or more. Anaemia can lead to delayed periods. Sometimes, menses does not occur for many mouths at a stretch. Deal with the anaemia first. Eat leafy vegetable and fruit but avoid eating refined flour products, sugar and milled rice as far as possible. Hot and cold hip baths can help. Yogic postures to relieve delayed menstruations include *Badha Konasana, Karna-pida Asana, Matsya Asana, Salamba Sirsh Asana, Supta-vajra Asana, Hal Asana.*

Disorders of Male and Women Genitalia

Urinary Calculi: Formation of stone in kidney, ureter or urethara generally due to calcium phosphate or oxalates.

Syphilis: A general disease due to sexual contact with infected opposite sex. Recommended yogic postures: *Kurm Asana, Bhunaman Asana, Upasita Kona Asana, Supta Vajra Asana, Ushtra Asana.*

Gonorrhoea: Causes by sexual contact with opposite sex in which there will be yellowish white discharge with pain. The disease spreads to other parts of body. The recommended yogic postures are similar to those as in case of syphilis.

Sterlity (Frigidity): A condition where in a women will be unable to conceive generally due to malfunctioning of fallopian tubes, uterus, ovaries, hormonal imbalance, anaemia, blood poisoning and malnutrition. This disorder of sexual weakness may hamper the function to give sex pleasure or sexual enjoyment. Recommend postures: *Paschimottan Asana, Sarvang Asana, Matsya Asana, Shav Asana, Sirsh Asana.*

Pain in Lower Belly: Due to weakness in pregnant women or due to infection in pelvic organs or urinary tract in men and women. Recommended postures: *Nauli Mudra, Ardh Chandra Asana, Yog Mudra.*

Scalding Urine: Causes burning sensation during urination, generally due to hyperacidity or malfunctioning of the kidneys. Recommended postures: *Salamba Sirsh Asana, Paschimottan Asana, Ardh Matsyendra Asana.*

Anaemia: Shortage of blood and sufficient iron in body is termed as anaemia. Pregnant women enter an anaemic condition in the 12th week and the condition reaches its climax in 32nd week. Recommended yogic exercises: *Pranayama e.g. Ujjayi* (energy renewing pranayama) and *Nadi-Sodhana* (alternate breathing), *Pachimottan Asana, Ardh Matsyendra Asana, Sarvang Asana, Shav Asana.*

Liver/Kidney Pain: These are common due to accumulation of acidity in gall bladder in women. Suddenly the pain starts from back and then passes to the right shoulder. In case of kidney pain, the pain starts from kidney and passes upward. Woman feels pain in the breasts. Recommended postures: *Matsya Asana, Sarvang Asana.*

Obstruction of Urine: Causes when uterus shifts its place and is pushed back developing pressure on the kidney affecting normal flow of urine accompanied by accumulation of blood or pus. As a result of obstruction in urine there is feeling of pain; inflammation and swelling in urethra and uterus. Recommended postures: *Ardha Sarvang Asana, Baddha Kona Asana, Matsya Asana, Karna-Pida Asana.*

Itching Pain in Vagina: The trouble is common among women those who have trouble of regular secretion. The itching usually causes due to semen remaining in the vagina after sexual intercourse. Too frequent sex should be avoided during pregnancy. Avoid too much scratching of gential organs and if the secretion touches the anus, itching pain and swelling spreads. Recommended postures: *Baddha Kona Asana, Yog Mudra, Mal Asana, Supta Vajra Asana, Pas Asana.*

Hydramnios: Develops in women in the 5th or 6th month after conception and sometimes results into miscarriage. In the uterus, there is a small membrane which is full of anamistic fluid in which the foetus develops. The membrane starts swelling resulting the placenta orifice gets closed due to inflammation and pain or the orifice of the placenta is closed. Perform very light yogic exercises as recommended by yoga experts.

Threatened Abortion: Have the symptoms of spotting i.e. a drop or two of blood oozing out of uterus. A complete rest is advised. Eat "Amla Murabba" wrapped in silver foil in the morning during throughout the period of pregnancy. Yoga exercises are not recommended.

Pain in Breasts during Lactation Period: The veins in the breast become engorged during lactation period. *Bhujang Asana* and *Dhanur Asana* are the recommended exercises.

Cystitis (Frequent Urination): The condition is common in the beginning of pregnancy or near the time of labour. Only light exercises for reproductive system are recommended.

Retention of Urine: This problem occurs during the third stage of pregnancy when the weight of the foetus presses upon the urethra. To relieve the presure, the doctor usually insert two finger into the vagina to lift the uterus little. Avoid strong diuretic in such condition. Recommended yogic postures: *Arhda Matsyendra Asana, Supta Vajra Asana*.

Vulvular Pruritis: Consists of intense itching in the genital tract during pregnancy. Avoid spices and cordiments. A warm water douche should be given and the genital tract should be painted with a solution of camphor mixed to rose water. Recommended postures: *Gomukh Asana, Ek Pada Uttan Asana, Yog Mudra*.

Cough, Cold and Bronchitis: It is also common among pregnants, generally due to pressure on lungs as a result of development of embryo. Sometimes, it develops into a whooping cough and cause danger of a miscarriage. Regular practice of *Kapalabhati, Pranayama, Neti* and *Dhuati* is an ideal remedy.

Vigour and Beauty: A sense of equilibrium revive the energy of body and one feels refreshed and charged with energy. Recommended postures: *Natraj Asana, Dhanur Asana, Viparitakarani, Kurm Asana, Vir-bhadra Asana, Uttan Asana.*

Nacturnal Emission: It is more common in male when there is seminal discharge during sleep usually due to mental tension, insecurity, frustration and seing sexy TV Programmes, adult movies and reading obsene literature. Recommended yogic postures *Baddha Kona Asana, Mula-badha, Yog mudra.*

Varicose Veins: It is caused due to lack of exercise, obesity and standing for long time, as a result blood circulation in the veins becomes slow causing congestion of blood. The valves in the veins become weak causing discomfort and pain in legs. Practice of inverted yogic exercises such as *Sirsh Asana, Salamba Sirsh Asana, Sarvang Asana, Viparitakarani* help the flow of blood towards the heart.

Apprehension of Miscarriage: The symptoms include pain or the slighest spotting (bleeding) by the expecant mother usually during the first trimester (upto 12 weeks) of pregnancy. A complete bed rest and a wet pack be placed on the pubes for an hour in the morning and evening. The process should be repeated on the dates the pregnant woman would have had her monthly period. After the third month the apprehension of a miscarriage will recede. Avoid yogic exercises strictly.

Childbirth in the Eighth Months: Usually the infant delivered in the eighth month does not survive. Deficiency of many natural salts including calcium affect the healthy growth of the child in the mother's womb due to abnormal development of foetus. The mother may suffer from weakness of the muscles which support the uterus and may suffer a miscarriage and even if there is a normal birth, the child is most likely to be sickly and weak. Calcium is found in leafy vegetables and milk in abudant quanities. Yogic postures which strengthen the reproductive organs are *Sirsh Asana, Salamba Sirsh Asana, Sarvang Asana, Paschimottan Asana, Supta Vajra Asana.*

Premature Ejaculation Among Men: It is a malfunctioning due to psychological reasons. The male is generally found to be sexually more aroused than the female who needs a bit of foreplay to be ready for sexual act. Too much of anticipation of the sex act, too much of excitment can lead to premature ejaculation giving a feeling of failure or lack of fulfilment which should follow the act of sexual intercourse. Yogic exercises to strengthen the nervous system are *Baddha Kona Asana, Mulabandha, Pachimottan Asana, Sirsh Asana, Salamba Sirsh Asana.*

Impotence (Sexual Weakness): It is the inability to perform the sexual act which may be partial or complete, temporary or permanent. The problem can be categorised into organic and psychological. Organic impotence may be caused by lesions of the external genitalia, such as light fore-skin of organs and disturbance of endocrine glands (thyroid glands or piturtary glands). Ignorance, fear, weakness of sexual desire are the psychological factors which give rise to impotence among male having been addicted to masturbation in adolescence or over indulged sex are another reason for the impotency. Consult a doctor in case of organic impotence. Sexual weakness hampers the functions of reproductive system: to perpetuate the species and to give pleasure to both partners due to sexual weakness. *Pranayama exercises (Kapalabhati followed by Bahya Kumbhaka)* with *bandhas* should be practiced daily. Yogic asanas such as *Sirsh Asana,*

Salamba Sirsh Asana, Sarvang Asana, Viparitakarani and Pachimottan Asana are beneficial to strengthen sex organs.

Yogic Posture Suitable for Disorders of Ovaries and Women Disorders

Ardha Matsyendra Asana (Simplified Yogi Matsyendra Posture): This asana is very useful to correct spinal deformities. It has beneficial effect on the gall bladder, spleen, kidneys and bowels. The back must remain straight during exercise and the spinal twist must be pefromed smoothly without exerting much force to the elbows.

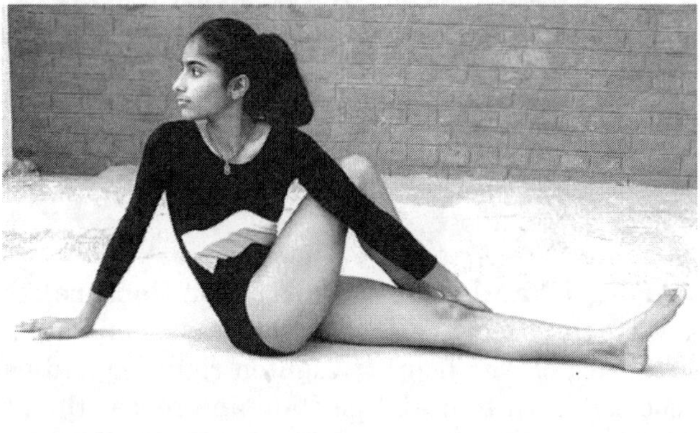

Matsyendra Asana (Yogi Matsyendra Asana): With the regular practice of Ardha Matsyendra Asana in the begining you may perform this asana effectively. To do Matsyendra Asana, sit, straighten the body, stretch both legs in front in parallel position and breathe normally. Fold the right leg at the knee by pulling it backward, the right thigh standing upward and the right side buttock raised up. At this stage, keep right leg standing. Now bring the whole right arm and hand. Now bring the whole right hand preferable touching the fingers on the back in a loose condition. Then turn the head chest and waist towards the right side twisting the body as much as possible exhaling. Stay in position for six to eight seconds, then unlock and return to the initial position of readiness, inhaling and exhaling deeply. Repeat the round to the other side. Matsyendra Asana has beneficial effect on the pancreas, adrenal, thyroid and sex glands. It fully activate the muscles of the stomach abdomen, intestine, pelvic, kidneys, spleen, liver, spinal cord and energizes and strengthens the body. The asana is especially good for diabetic patients.

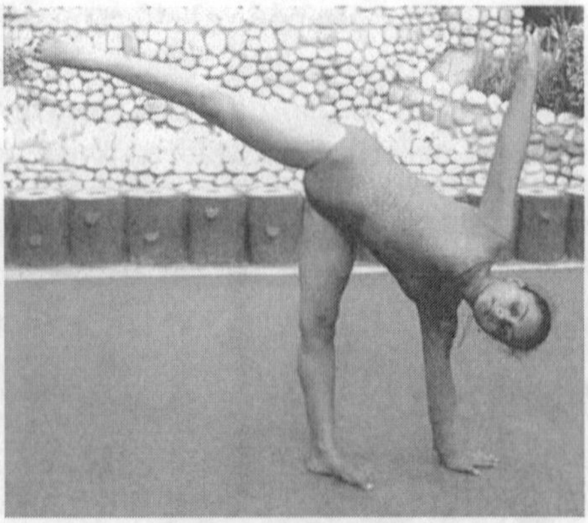

Ardha Chandrasana (Half- Moon Posture): Spread legs two to three feet apart, arms side ways. Bend right knee, raise left leg off the floor, straighten right leg and balance the body. Return to initial position and repeat the posture on other side. This posture softens up the spinal column and pelvic region. It slims down the hips, waist and lower back.

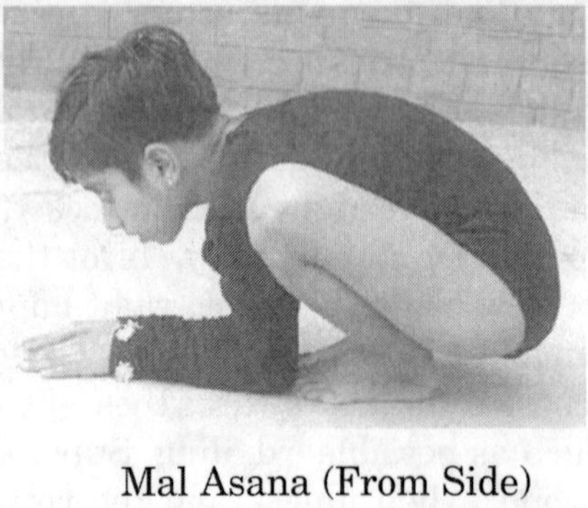

Mal Asana (From Side)

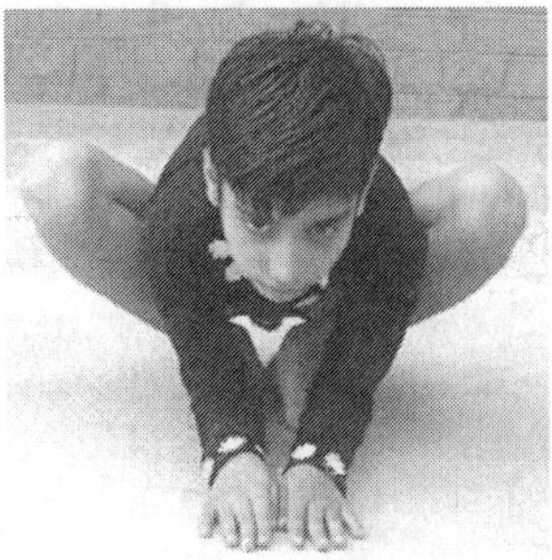

Mal Asana (From Front)

Mal Asana (Garland Posture): This posture tones up abdominal organs, soothes backache, cures all menstruation disorders in women, elongates muscles of the back and renders the ankel flexible.

Yogic Posture for Female Diseases

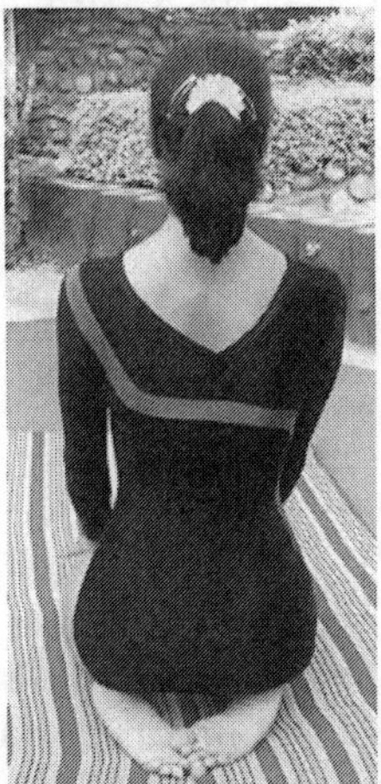

Manduk Asana (Frog Position): Sit on your folded legs, breathing normally, fold your left foot on left side and right foot on your right side. Supporting the body weight separate knees moving the left knee further to the left side and right knee to the right side, trying to separate them as much as you can do comfortably. Look in front, breath normally, stay in this position for 8 to 12 seconds. Return to the sitting position. Rest for six to eight seconds, then repeat the asana two to four times. This asana is very effective asana for reducing the weight of the thighs, hips and abdominal areas leaving good impact on the muscles and nerves of the lower portion of the body. The posture enhances sexual potentiality, corrects disorders of the reproductive system, cures piles, strengthens the digestive system and allows greater blood supply to the stomach.

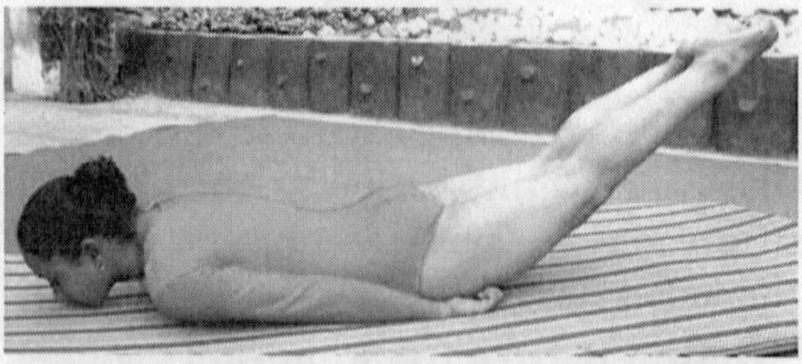

Salabh Asana with both legs

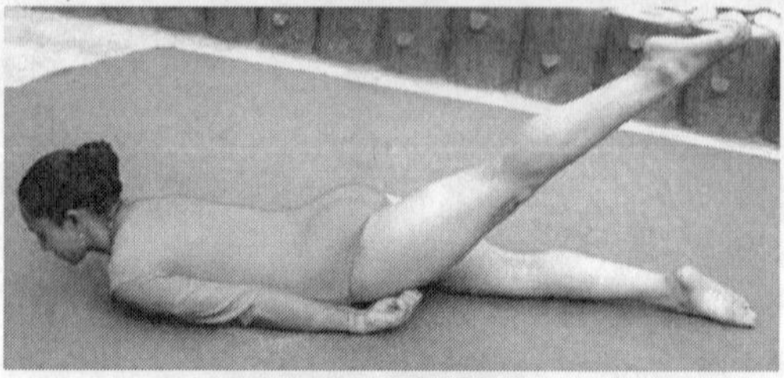

Salabh Asana with one leg

Salabh Asana (Locust Posture): Lie on stomach with chin or forehead touching the ground. Stretch the arms on sides of the body. Inhale, tense the arms, clench the fists tightly. Raise the legs as high as possible. Hold the position for few seconds retaining breath. Hold for sometime then exhale and lower the legs. Repeat lying on stomach. Repeat exercises three to four times. The posture has excellent effect on the muscles of the back, arms and abdomen. It leaves beneficial effects on digestive organs, cures constipation and cleanse the kidneys. In case of difficulty to raise both legs, practice with the simplified posture *'Ardh-Salabh Asana'* which has benefits to similar to Salabh asana.

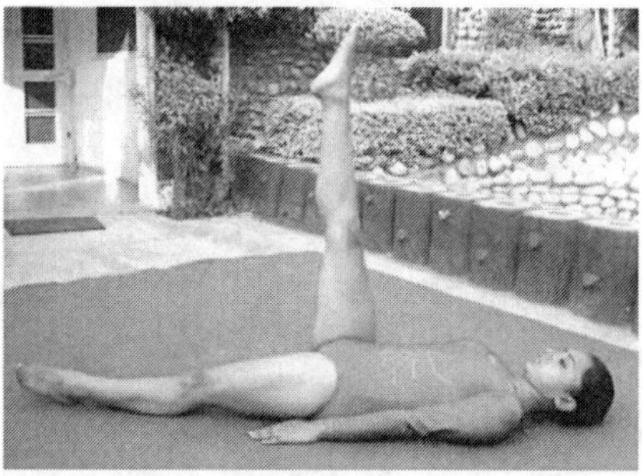

Ek Pada Uttana Asana: Women suffering from white vaginal discharge and menstrual disorders have a curative effect with the regular practice of this asana. It tones up the muscles of the sex-glands and enhances potentiality. To practice this asana, lie down on your back, palms near the body and heels together. Breathe normally, look straight upward. Let the body remain loose. Now raise one leg upward slowly towards the sky (inhaling) in a perpendicular position without straining, twisting and turning the hips and waist while lifting the leg. Hold for six seconds retaining the breathe and lower the leg towards, the floor exhaling. When the leg comes to the floor, rest for 6 to 8 seconds and repeat the same process with other leg. Start with four rounds. This exercise cures asthmatics, brings flexibility to hip joints, corrects disorders of stomach and intestine, removes wind troubles and gastric condition of the digestive system.

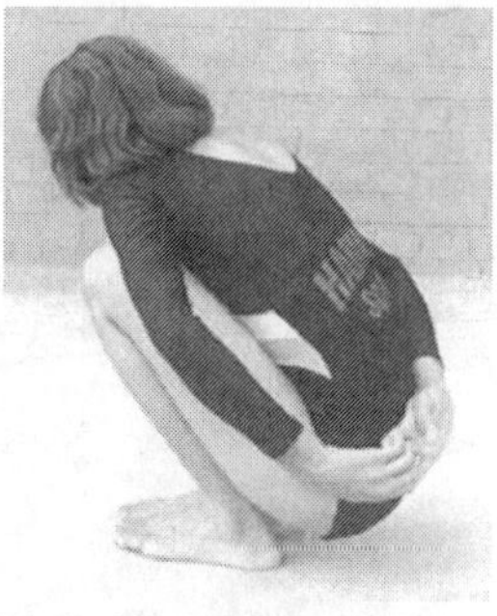

Pas Asana

Pas Asana (The Chord Posture): This posture is beneficial to spinal column, liver, spleen and pancreas. It gets rid of fat around waist and stomach. Pas Asana relieves women from delayed menstruation and itching pain in vagina.

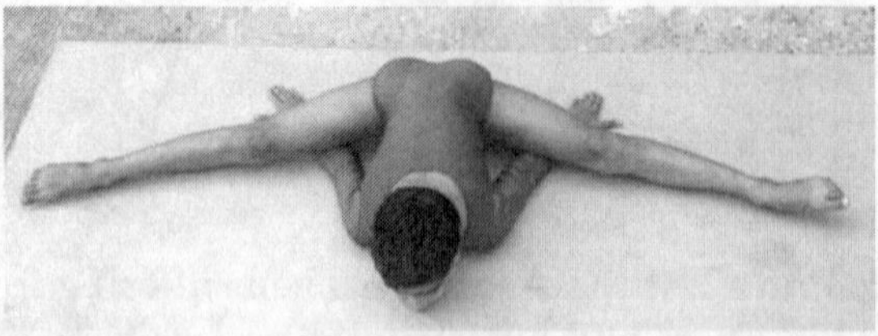

Kurm Asana (Tortoise Posture): This yogic posture has a beneficial effect on the spinal column and nervous system. It tones up abdominal organs and the whole body is charged with energy.

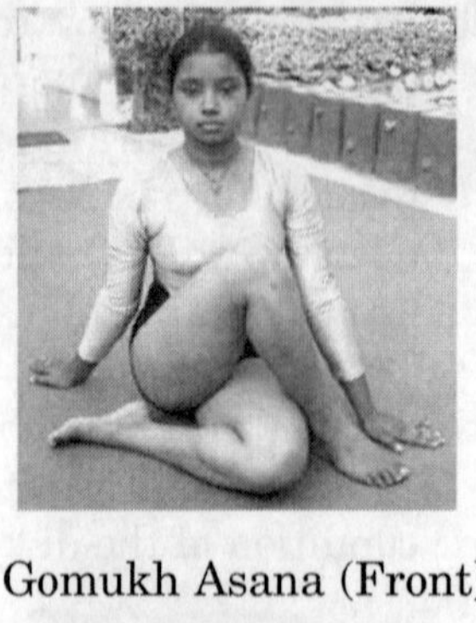

Gomukh Asana (Front)

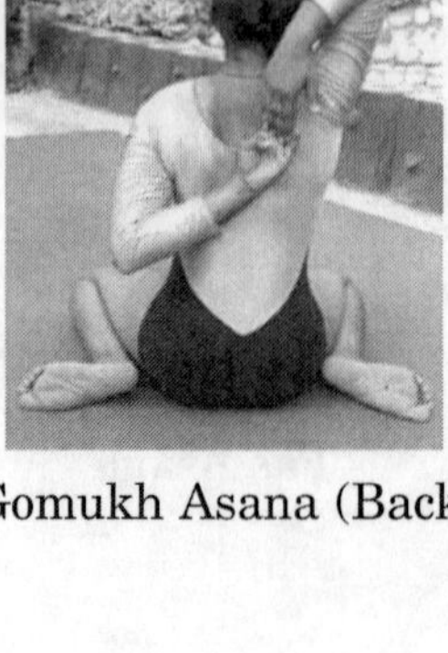

Gomukh Asana (Back)

Gomukh Asana (Cowhead Posture): Sit on the floor. Fold left leg in and right leg over the left leg so that one knee lies over the other. Take left arm on the back placing left hand between shoulder blades. Now take right hand behind on the back and hook fingers with the fingers of left hand. Interchange the position of your legs and arms. This posture relieves cramps in the calves, tones up the joint muscles and nerves, activates muscles and nerves of entire body, restores the synovial fluid (a joint fluid in the body), strengthens the bones, helps bust development and strengthens the lungs and heart.

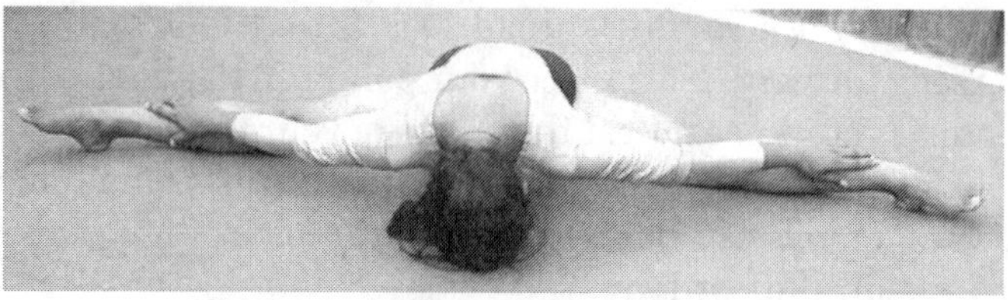

Upavista Kona Asana: Upavista means seated and Kona means angle. This asana keeps joints, muscles, organs and nerves strong and healthy. To do this asana, wide your legs as much as you can sideways, one leg at a time. Tighten the muscles of your legs and keep toes pointing upwards. Sit erect. Now hook big toes with your index and middle fingers. Bend forward and rest your forehead or chin on the floor. Do not bend your knees. This exercise improves circulation in the pelvic region and makes hamstring muscles elastic. The asana is especially good for mensutration disorders of women, strengthens genital organs, increses sex power. This asana can be performed on single leg also. Sit in Upavista Kona Asana. Rotate waist to left, hold your left foot with both hands. Rest your chin or forehead on your left knee. Now rotate your waist to right side. Finally return to initial position.

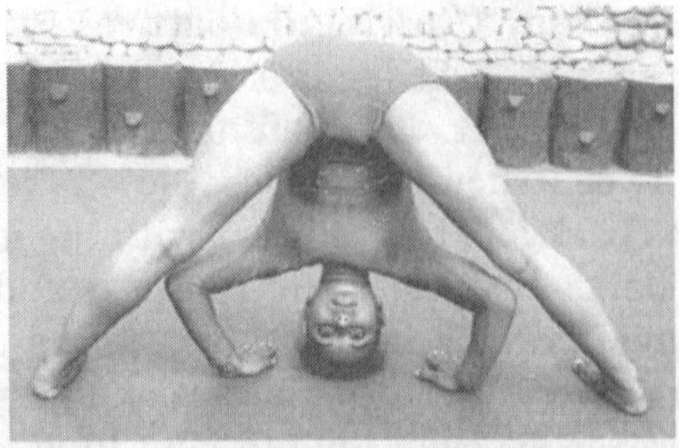

Parasarita Pada Uttana Asana: Parasarita means spread. Pada means legs. Uttana means intense. Beneficial incase of suffering from dysmenorrhoea. To practice this asana, stand straight, spread legs 3 to 4 feet apart, toes pointing forward. Now place your palms on the floor without bending your knees. Rest the crown of your head on the floor. Hold for sometime, then raise your head. This asana removes fatigue, improves arches, relieves cramps in the calves and cures genital disorders.

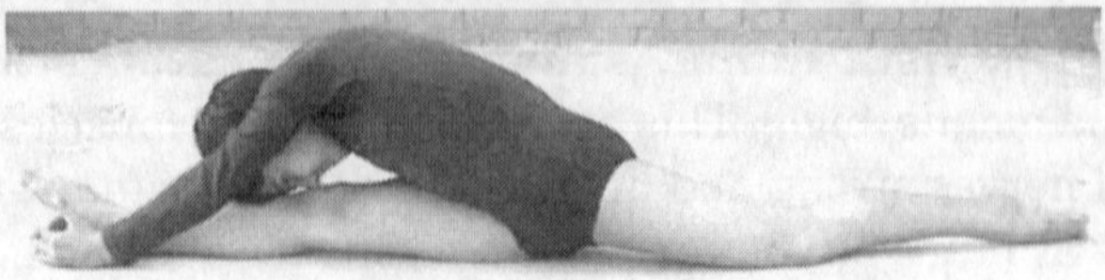

Bhunaman Asana (Sideward Leg-stretch, Head to Ground): This posture allows the leg muscles to the elongated, spinal column stretched, sympathic column stretched and sympathic nerves massaged. It strengthens genital organs.

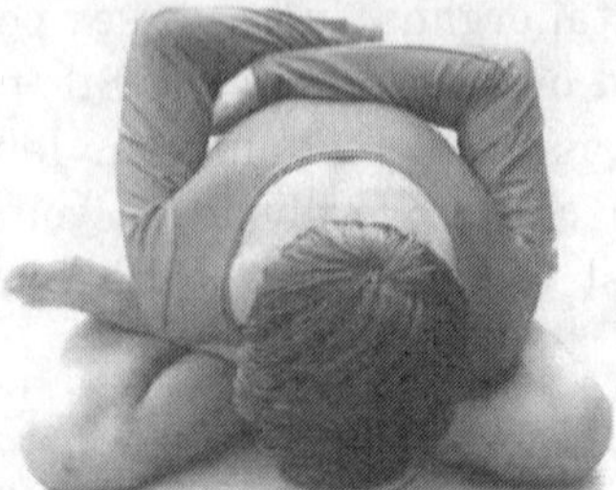

Ardh Badha Padma Asana (Toe-hold Lotus Posture): This posture cures premature separation of placenta, common disorder among pregnant women. This asana helps relieve the trouble. Sit in Padma Asana. Breathe out sharply and bring left hand behind your back and catch hold of your left big toe with right hand. Look straight. This is **Ardha Baddha Padma Asana**. Now bend forward resting your forhead on the ground. Repeat posture 3 to 4 times with 20 to 30 counts each. This posture is effective against slow bowel movement and renders the whole body supple. It develops the thoracic cage and improves respiration and strengthens the shoulders.

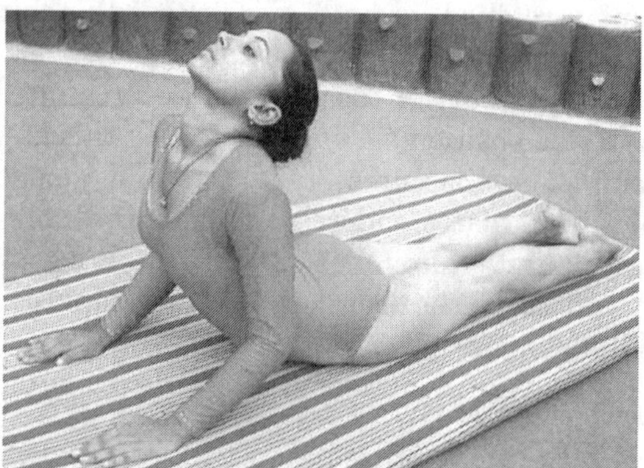

Bhujang Asana (Cobra Posture): Lie on your stomach. Place your palms to the sides of the chest. Inhale. Raise your head and trunk slowly leaning back as far as possible without raising the abdominal region. Hold for few seconds, then exhale slowly. Repeat this exercise two to three times. This asana helps to cure all female disorders and strengthen the muscles of breasts (The asana is beneficial for under developed breasts).

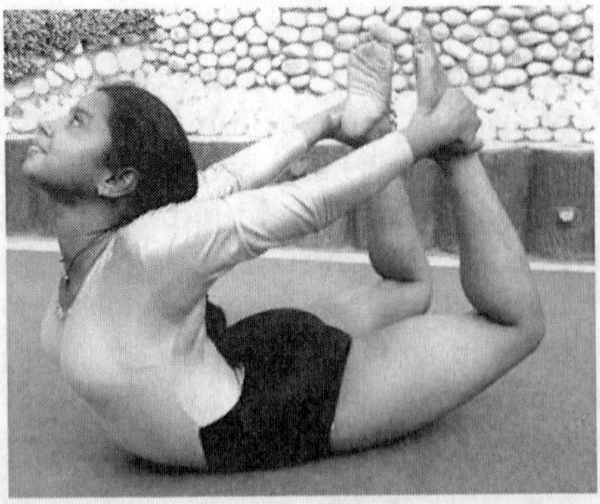

Dhanur Asana (Bow Posture): Lie on stomach. Keep your arms stretched on both sides. Rest the chin on the ground and take the ankles in the hands. Now raise the legs, head and upper part of the body while arching the back. Remain in this position as long as possible this asana tones the abdominal organs, cures irregular or faulty menstruation in females, stimulates endocrine glands, prevents fat from forming around stomach and hips, has curative and corrective effects on the disorders of joints, spinal cord, lungs, chest and abdomen.

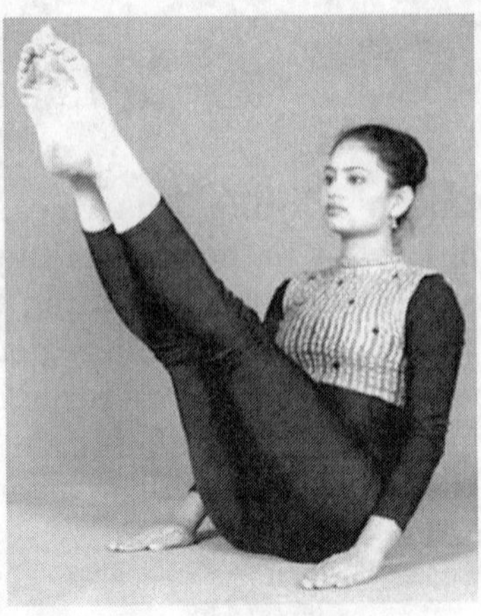

Vajroli Mudra (Boat Posture): This balancing pose strengthens thighs and abdominal muscles. The asana rids the digestive organs of toxins and helps to develop the sex will-power in men and women between the age of 25 to 40.

Postures for Pregnant Women

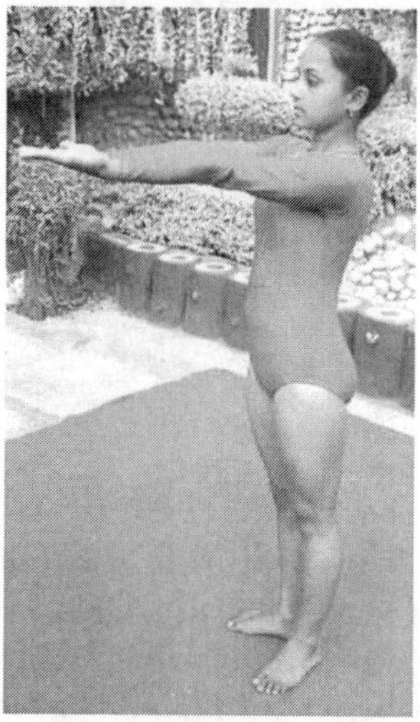

Position-1

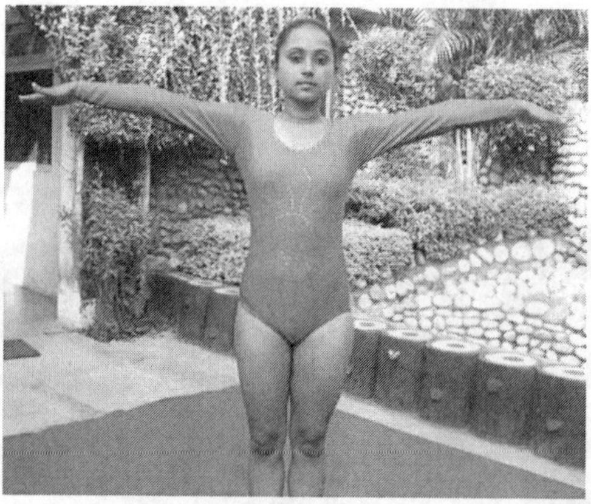

Position-2

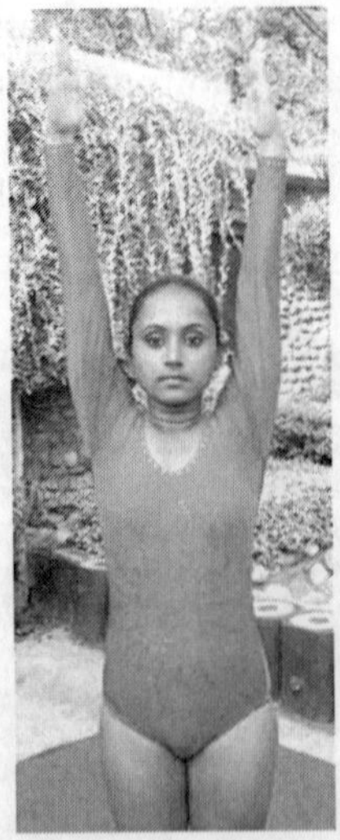

Position-3

Tara Asana: This posture has three positions. Stand straight, raise your arms opposite. Hold for 10 to 15 seconds. Now raise your arms straight over the head. Hold for 10 to 15 seconds. Finally bring both hands on sides parallel to the ground. Hold for 10 to 15 seconds. This is a light exercise done during pregnancy which keep the body in order. It has strengthening effect upon lungs, chest and respiration system. The exercise corrects disorders of asthmatics, pain in the shoulder joints and helps those who wish to add a few inches to their height.

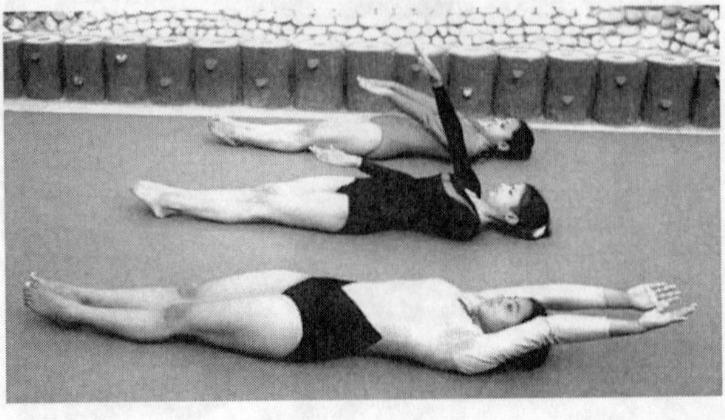

Hasta Parshav Asana: Lie on your back, arms on sides. Raise arms and rotate in clockwise in circle behind the head inhaling. Repet the exercise four time and gradually increase to ten times. It is an ideal exercise for strengthening the muscles of arms and shoulders.

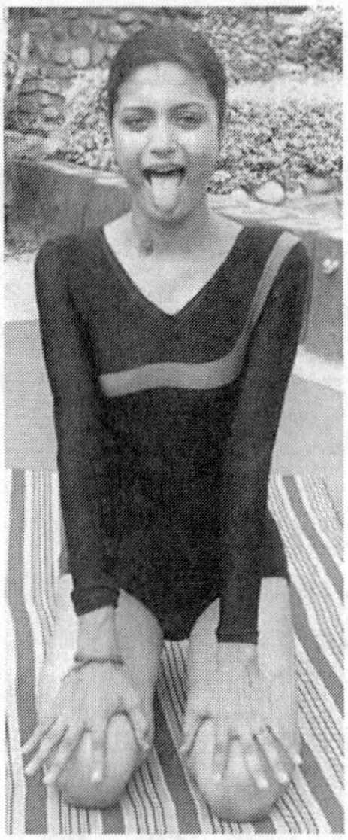

Simha Asana: This asana refreshed the whole body during early and middle stage of pregnancy. If you feel uncomfortable in Padma Asana, sit in Vajra Asana. Place your palms on the floor in front and raise your buttocks. Now move buttocks down towards floor. Open your mouth wide. Stretch your tongue out towards your chin. Gaze at the tip of your nose or between the eyebrows. Begin with two rounds daily during the first trimester of pregnancy and gradually increase to four rounds during the second trimester of the pregnancy. This asana helps get rid of bad breath and cure throat troubles. It makes the lower spine elastic and has good effect on the respiratory system. This exercise is also very beneficial for children and housewives.

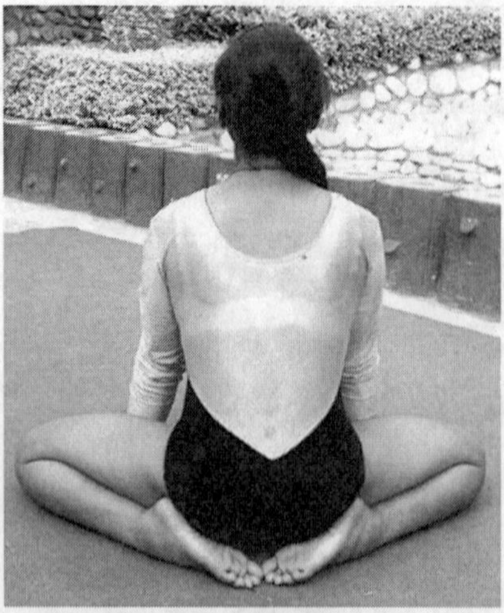

Vira Asana (Warrior Posture): To practice this asana, sit on the floor with both legs bent back. Your hips must rest on the floor between the feets. Sit erect looking straight. This is Vira Asana posture I. Now spread your knees wide apart and join big toes. Bend forward and rest your forehead on the floor stretching your arms. Draw your shoulders back and sit straight. This is Vira Asana posture II. This asana is beneficial for the pregnant women which removes pain, cramps and fatigue in the legs. It makes knee joint flexible and strong, corrects flat feet, strengthens ankels and aids digestion.

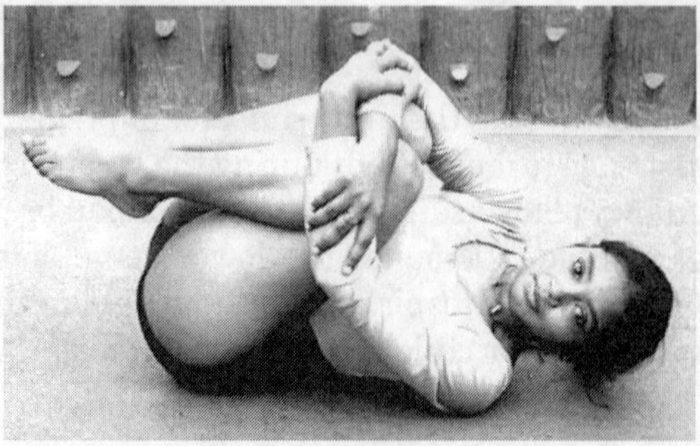

Pawan Mukta Asana: The practice of Pawan Mukta-Asana strengthens the upper part of the body if performed during pregnancy. The secreationing of hormones increases. This asna relieves lines and wrinkles on waist, abdomen. It tones up muscles of abdomen and intestines, cures constipation and gastric trouble, corrects malfunctioning of the stomach. Practice of this posture helps uterus come to original place during childbirth. Pawan Mukta Asana can be done in standing position or lying on the back on the floor. Stand up straight keeping both hands hanging down. Lift one knee up towards the chest. Pull the knee up towards the chest without any pull on the ankle. Stand firmly on the other leg. Stay in this position for 6 to 8 seconds, then release the knee on the floor. Rest for 6 to 8 seconds and repeat the exercise with the other leg. In case of difficulty in practising this asana in standing position, do it lying on the back—the method of practice remains the same as in the standing position.

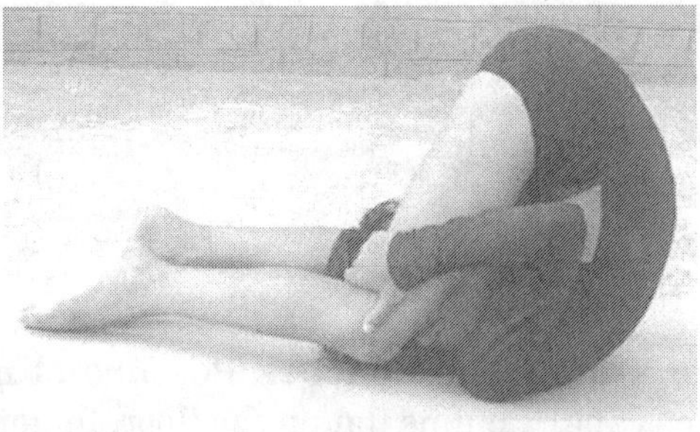

Karna-Pida Asana: Helps relieve digestive problems, keeps the spinal column supple and healthy, revitalizes the nerves and muscles of back, removes exhaustion and fatigue quickly, relieves obstruction of urine, prevents fat from forming on the stomach, hips and waist. To do Karna-Pida Asana, complete the posture of Hala Asana, Now bend your knees and rest then on the ground close to your ears. Rest your arms on your calves.

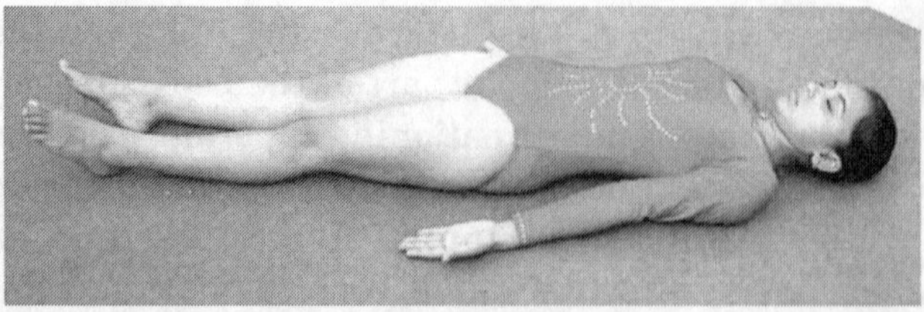

Shava Asana: Relaxes all body muscles, nerves, the organs of the bodily system, gain strength and restore normal health. Those who feel lack of energy, tiredness, fatigue and lack of vitality will find this asana to provide energy and strength. Make Shav Asana at the end of all postures. In case of hypertension and heart troubles, Shav Asana should be performed singly for longer period. To do Shava Asana, lie on your back keeping whole body loose, breathing normally. Do not use pillow under your head. Keep your eyes closed, bring your mental attention towards the toes. This asana is especially beneficial for those suffering from anemia.

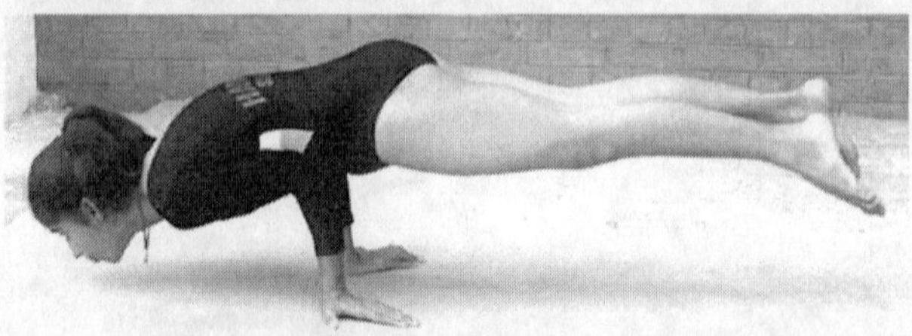

Mayur Asana (The Peacock Posture): Kneel on the ground, knees apart, palms flat on the floor, fingers pointing towards the face, bringing the elbows under the abdomen just under the navel. Lean forward to touch the ground with forehead and stretch out the legs behind raising the face and head and keeping the body (Parallel to the ground). Stay balanced on the arms as long possible, then lie down on the stomach, relax for sometime breathing normally and repeat. The posture increases supply of blood to the digestive organs and cures constipation. It tones up the abdominal muscles, brings the body into equilibrium, strengthen the muscles and forearms. The asana helps to regenerate energy in the body.

Mula Bandha Asana (Contraction of the Pelvic and anal Muscles): In sanskrit word Mula means roots or source and Bandha means contraction. The posture is similar to Paschimottan Asana in which the breath is held contracting the ring of muscles around the anus causing the whole of the pelvic region to contract. Repeat exercise several times always perform this posture with the lungs empty. If carried out incorrect exercise, it can lead to chronic constipation and faulty digestive system. This asana stimulates the muscles around the anus and lower part of the trunk. It regenerates sexual glands. Very useful for those teenagers suffering from nacturnal emission.

7

Psychological Problems of Child and Teenagers

Faulty learning is the main cause of faulty behaviour, which plays havoc with the development of the child's personality. The following are the faulty behaviours of child and teenagers:

Thumb Sucking: It is a normal phenomenon in early infancy generally due to hunger. If after the age of five, child sucks his thumb consult a child psychologist. A child addicted to thumb-sucking may harm his teeth—the upper teeth will protrude forward while the lower tend to be drawn inwards or backwards.

Teeth Grinding: It is a harmless habit. In older child and teenages, teeth grinding may be accompanied by talking during sleep due to tension. The behaviour reflects that the child is not able to assimilate adequately and manage his tensions of the day. *Sirsh Asana, Shav Asana* and *Viparitakarani* are recommended yogic postures to relieve tension.

Nail biting (Onychophagia): Helps a child as well as a teenager to get relief from pressure or anxiety.

Picking the Nose: These are the signs of tension. Better to understand the cause of tension. Recommended yogic postures *Sirsh Asana, Shav Asana* and *Vipritakaran.*

Biting the lips: It is common among children and the teenagers due to tension. Recommended yogic postures *Viparitakarani* and *Sirsh Asana*.

Twisting strand of hair: A child or teenager prones to this behaviour due to psychological factors. Recommended yoga postures: *Yog Mudra, Vakra Asana* and *Sarvang Asana*.

Tics (Habit Spasm): These are the signs of emotional disturbance which occur frequently between the age of 6 to 15 some example of fics include shoulder shrugging, eye blinkign, neck twisting and dry coughing. These symptoms are seen as a result of tense among children (between age 6 to 10 years) and teenagers due to strict parents, scolding attitude to them and teasing and nagging by companions in the educational institutes worsen the condition. Recommended yoga postures include *Mayur Asana, Seta-bhandu Sarvang Asana*.

Prevented appetite: Usually as a result of deficiency of calcium and iron or a nutrition cause when a child develops the habit to eat mud, sand, wall paint, animal dropping, grass wool, ashes, faeces, coal and so on. Keep watch on your child more carefully and engage him busy in activities. If a child eats rubbish, he is likely to develop intestinal illness. Consult a child specialist.

Temper Tantrums: Oftenly, hunger and fatigue result in outbursts of temper. If a tantrum does occur, it may be sparked off by a refusal to each change clothes and go to school. Avoid to scold the child for feeling angry, that makes children more aggressive. *Ardha-Matsyendra Asana* and *Hal Asana* are recommended postures for the problem.

Fear: Mostly children and teenage female are afraid of something or the other—it may be snake, cat, dog, a thunder storm the dark or deep water. Usually these fears are transitory and can disappear once the source of the fear has been identified. Do not tell frightening sotries or allow to see horror movies to your children and teenagers. Fears are often cause by lack of confidence. Yogic Asanas such as *Vakra Asana, Paschimottan Asana, Urdhva Hasta Asana* and *Uddiyana* are beneficial to treat fear.

Destructiveness: Children in adolescent can be destructive carelessly and unintentionally or deliberately. He breaks a toy or destroy things despite warnings from the elders. Frustration is the basic cause of this trouble for which practice of *Yog Mudra, Hal Asana, Sarvang Asana* and *Vakra Asana* are beneficial yogic postures.

Stammering (Shuttering): A speech disorder that involves blocking or repetition of, or sometimes a struggle usually exhibits a few behaviours like blinking, jerking of hand, jerking of arms, movement of the lips, frowning, swallowing, clenching of fists and stamping of feet etc. The main causes of this disorder are due to a stressful situation that leads to severe feeling of inadequate self-consciousness, anxiety fear and tension. Shuttering results in shyness and sensitiveness in a child or adult. Following are few treatments:

1. **Assertion Training:** It is a behaviour therapy procedure which attempts to help a person express more easily his thoughts, wishes, beliefs and feelings of resentment or approval.
2. **Aversive Conditioning:** It is use of harmful stimuli to punish unwanted behaviour.
3. **Desensitization:** It is a therapeutic process by which reaction to traumatic experiences are reduced. Recommended Yogic postures include *Bak Asana, Prasarita Pada-Uttan Asana, Uttana Asana, Adho-Mukha Shavana Asana, Sirsh Asana, Supt Vajra Asana.*

Enuresis (Bed-Wetting): It refers to the habitual involuntary discharge of urine, more common at night or may also occur during day time while in sleep. Among older children or adults those suffering from enuresis often occur in conjunction with dreams imaging that he or she is urinating are the causes attributed to bed wetting. Do not take liquid or give to the child two hours before going to bed. Faulty learning or lack of toilet trainign, personal immaturity associated with emotional problems, disturbed family atmosphere leading to sustained anxiety, urinary tract infection, worm infestation are the prominent causes. Yogic Asanas i.e. *Vakra Asana, Paschimottan Asana* and *Uddiyana* are recommended.

Sleep Walking (Somnambulism): Some children as well as adult experience regular or periodic sleepwalking episodes. In this condition children go to sleep in a normal manner but get up during second or third hour of their sleep and may walk to another room or outside. Such episodes usually last from 15 minutes to about an hour and the person in sleep returns to bed; but in the morning he/she is usually unawair of anything. The causes of sleep-walking are not fully understood. Infact, sleep-walking is related to some anxiety arousing situation. Psychotherapy (the treatment of mental disorders by pscyhological methods) has been proved useful for the treatment of sleep-walking. Reduce distress the yogic ways by regular practice of Asanas such as *Yog Mudra, Vakra Asana, Trikona Asana*.

Phobic Neurosis: It is a persistent fear of some objects or situations. Some common phobias include Acrophobia (fear of high places), Agoraphobia (fear of open places), Algophobia (fear of pain), Astraphobia (fear of storms), thunder and lightenings, claustrophobia (fear of closed places), Hematophobia (fear of blood), Mysophobia (fear of contamination), Monophobia (fear of lonliness), Nycrophobia (fear of crowds), Pathophobia (fear of disease), Pyrphobia (fear of fire), syphilophobia (fear of syphilis) and zoo phobia (fear of animals). Recommended Yogic Postures include *Vakra Asana* and *Paschimottan Asana*.

Hyperactivity: A common child/adult disorder characterized by over-activity, restlessness and distractability. Hyperactive children suffer from a disease called Hyperkinetic Child Syndrome disorder. The specific causes of Hyperactivity is not known as there are several psychological factors that could lead to this disorder: generally suffering from premature births, minimum brain dysfunction and development of central nervous system. Behaviour therapy is useful in hyperactivity among children and teenager. Excessive intake of tea, coffee, beverages, chocolates, additives and foods with artificial flavour should be avoided. Yogic exercises such as *Padma Asana, Sukhasana, Viparitakarani, Natraj Asana* and *Shava Asana* are recommended incase of hyperactivity.

Shyness and Withdrawal: Children, mostly female sex tend towards seclusiveness, timidity and inability to form close interpersonal relationship. It occurs in those children not given a chance to mix with another children and adults, over protectiveness by parents, have inherited shyness from parents, repeated experience of failure, stemming from poor learning skills and separation from mother for longer time. Such children should be allowed to go out to visit friends and to do things for themselves. Yoga postures such as *Vakra Asana, Pachimottan Asana, Yog Mudra* and *Hal Asana* are beneficial in this condition.

School Phobia: It is common not only among school children but also the teenagers are reluctant because of acute fear associated with it. The main causes of phobia are lengthy and frequent separation of child from the parents, fear of a teacher, threats by class mates, improper dress, feelings of insecurity, mental subnormality and physical illness. *Vakra Asana* and *Paschimottan Asana* are the yogic exercise which help to relieve from this problem.

Masturbation: Many times children and teenagers of both sexes are seen rubbing their thighs or play with their sex organs and find a pleasure. A regular practice of *Setu-*

bandha Sarvang Asana and *Yog Mudra* help to relieve it. Around the age of three a child becomes aware that he is a boy or she is a girl. If a male child sees his sister undressed he becomes aware that something extra which his sister does not have. Similary, a female child is aware that she lacks the appendage which a male child has. Children in the habit of excessive of sex organs, you can, however give the child plenty to do with hands. Give him toys to play which directs his attention elsewhere. When a child is naked, the adults start teasing him, this type of attitude makes the child terribly conscious of his sex. The feeling of guilt towards the sex organs is not a healthy attitude. These attitudes carry on in adult life and may create psycho-sexual problem. In rare educational institutes sex education is a part of curriculum. It is the best that matters related to sex education are discussed with the child by the parents themselves or a senior member of the family. Adolescent child need to be given correct information about sex. Tell your daughter about menstruation before it starts. Similarly tell your son about nocturnal emissions (wet dreams). Recommended yogic postures: *Baddha Kona Asana, Adho-Mukha Shavana Asana, Uttana Asana, Parasarita Pada Uttan Asana*.

Mental Retardation: It is a state of arrested or incomplete development of mind. Mentally retared children should be advised to practice *Vir Bhadra Asana, Sarvang Asana, Adho-Mukha Shavana Asana, Uttana Asana, Parasarita Pada Uttan Asana* and *Matsaya Asana*.

Correct Grooming of a Child: The following yogic exercises enhance grooming and posture of a child:

Vriksha Asana, Urdhva Hasta Asana, Setu-bandha Sarvang Asana, Garuda Asana, Utthita Trikona Asana, Parivritta Trikona Asana, Virbhadra Asana, Uttana Asana, Sirsh Asana, Sirsh Salamba Asana, Sarvang Asana, Hal Asana, Padma Asana, Matsya Asana, Yog Mudra, Ardha Baddha Padma Asana, Paschimottan Asana, Urdhva

Dhanur Asana, Bak Asana, Parasarita Pada Uttan Asana and Adho Muka Shavana Asana.

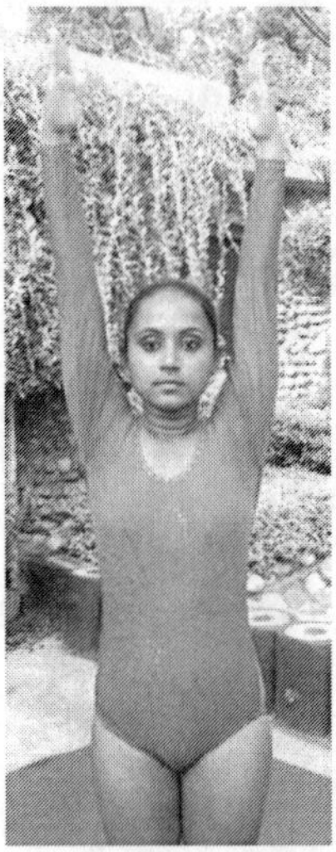

Tada Asana: Tada means mountain, stand straight joining your feet, tighten your knees big toes touching each other. Extend your arms downwards with palms facing your thighs. Look straight ahead and inhale exhale normally.

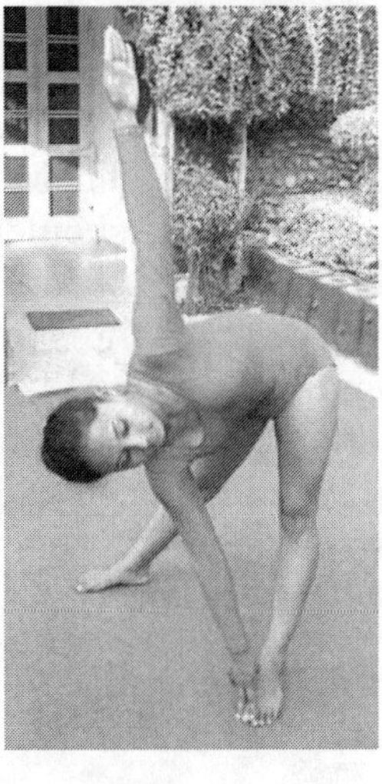

Trikona Asana (Traingle Posture): Stand with the legs apart. Inhale whilst raising the arms. Rotate waist, begin to exhale until the fingers of the right hand touches the ground. The arms should form a vertical line with the face turned upwards. Now stand up inhaling at the same time and perform the same movement to the other hands. Finish the exercise by exhaling. This posture tones up the muscles in the back, hips and legs. It makes the entire body strong and elastic.

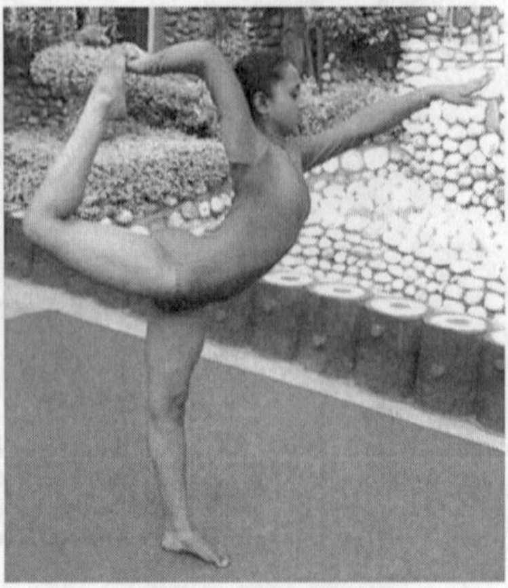

Nataraja Asana (Natraja Posture): Natraj posture is dedicated to Lord Shiva. As a cosmic dancer, Shiva is called the God of Dance. This posture generates vigour, vitality, potency, flexibility to the limbs, shoulders and hip joints, strengthens the major bones of the body, enhances digestive power, leaves good effect upon the spine, removes spinal rigidity and pain, improves eyesight. Perform Asana as shown in the illustration. Stay in this position for eight to ten seconds and keep breathing normal. Perform posture on both legs-left and then on right leg. Make 4 to 6 rounds daily.

8

The Magic of Herbs

Aloe Extract: A popular botanical recognized for centuries as having beneficial medicinal properties including antibiotic, anti-inflammatory and wound healing. Aloe vera is used in cosmetic preparations due to its moisturizing, soothing and calming properties. It is excellent for dry and sensitive skins as well as for the treatment of sun-burns and other minor burns, insect bites and skin irritations. Aloe extract is obtained from the aloe vera leaves and is also referred to as aloe vera gel. Aloe vera juice is the diluted version of aloe vera gel.

Aloe vera is an emollient and film forming gum resin with hydrating, softening, healing, anti-microbial and anti-inflammatory properties having strong moisturizing ability. It penetrates the skin, supplying moisture directly to the tissue, moisture regulation and absorb UV light. It has relaxing effect on the skin, making it beneficial for sensitive, sunburned and sun-exposed skins. In addition, it is found to be an effective component in emulsions formulated for dry skin. Apparently, aloe vera also has a synergistic effect when used in conjunction with other anti-inflammatory substances. It increases the blood supply to the area of application. Aloe vera is constituted of about 95 per cent water and the remaining constituents include minerals, polysaccharides, amino acids and carbohydrates.

Alder: This herb plant grows near water, where it can be assured of moist soil. It is commonly found on river-sides and marshy ground. Shiny oval leaves of alder enjoy the reputation of curing dropsical conditions caused by disorders of the renal system. The infusion may be used as a lotion for cooling sore, tired feet and prevent fatigue when walking.

Almond: Ground almond are extensively used in face masks. It is good for nourishing and cleansing. The Almond seeds contain 45 to 56 per cent oil, which is known as "badam rogan". The oil is very rich and used in various preparations for skin care.

Angelica: A large aromatic plant has drowny, triangular leaves and white or more rarely pale-purple flowers. Angelica in both extract and essential oil form, is a herb for the digestion, bringing swift relief from flatulence, colic and heart-burn. An infusion made from the leaves and chopped stem is a tonic, detoxifying and purifying agent. Principal constituents of this herb are volatile oil (about 1%), valeric acid, angelic acid, sugar and a resin called anglecin. Angelica extract is made from the seeds and the roots. It provides an excellent gargle for the treatment of sore tonsils and throats. The plant is used to flavour many alcoholic drinks.

Arnica Extract: A botanical credited with wide variety of properties such as antiseptic, astringent, anti-microbial, anti-inflammatory, anti-coagulant, circulatory, healing and stimulating. Arnica extract is also considered excellent for an acne condition, is effective in gels and creams designed to treat damaged, reddened or tired skin. The extract is obtained from the flowers. Repeated applications may produce severe inflammation in its use on sensitive skins.

Avocado Oil: It is obtained from the ripe avocado fruit and expressed from the seeds. Rich and nourishing with high vitamin contents. The pulp is used in face masks and the oil in nourishing creams. Avocado oil can function as an emollient and as a carrier oil in cosmetic preparations. Its skin-benefiting properties include bactericidal and soothing, particularly to sensitive skin. Avocado oil may increase the collagen of connective tissue and keeps the skin moist and smooth in addition to having the treatment for minor skin conditions. In cosmetic formulations, it helps to stabilize oil in water emulsions and effectively used in cleansing creams, moisturizers, lipsticks, make-up bases, bath oils, sunscreen and suntan preparations. Avocado oil enjoys the highest penetration rate among other oils such as corn, soyabean, olive and almond. It consist constituents such as oleic, linoleic and linolenic acid, palmitic and palmitoleic acid, lecithin, phytosterol, cartinoids and a high concentration of vitamins A, D and E.

Balm (Melissa officinalis): A fragrant woodland plant with dark green wrinkled leaves and small creamy flowers. It helps in the treatment of eczema, dry skin and acne formulations and products for blemished or sensitive skins. The herbs is credited with calming, soothing, healing, antispasmodic, tightening, anti-bactericidal and circulation-stimulating properties. Its effectiveness is due to the constituents such as citral, citronella, linalol, geraliol and aldehydes. Balm mint oil has sedative, antiplasmodic and antiseptic effect.

Balsam Peru: It is a botanical attributed to strong medicinal actions, recommended for curing scabies and skin diseases. The herb is considered antibacterial and sulphur based recommended for use on acne skin and eczema.

Basil (Tulsi): An a romantic herb with white flowers and oval - shaped, shiny leaves. Medicinally, basil is a potent tonic whose effect is both stimulant and nervine. It is particularly good at arresting morning and travel sickness besides, an effective skin tonic, application in acne preparations and rich in Vitamin C. Basil oil is often used as a carrier oil and its properties include stimulating, tonic, purifying and anti-microbial.

Babchi: A well-known medicinal herb, used as laxative and anthelmintic (antiparasite). Seeds of babchi cure leucoderma (white patches) on the skin.

Babool (Kikar): Used to clean the teeth. The leaves help relieve prolapse of rectum. Useful in cough, asthama and pittuisis. Decoction can help prevent threatened abortion.

Blackberry (Jamun): Berries are not only delicious but good for anaemia conditions as well. The leaves are mildly aperient and accredited with sound tonic virtues. An infusion is made and applied externally as a lotion to cure psoriasis and scaly conditions of the skin.

Blackberry extract is regarded as excellent for its astringent and tonic properties due to the high tannin content of the root, bark and the leaves. The leaf extract accredited with sound tonic virtues can be beneficially used for acne conditions. A standard infusion is made, which can be applied externally as a lotion to cure psoriasis and scaly conditions of the skin.

Betony (Chhitran Parni): A purple-flowered plant, is a natural pain killer, especially good for headaches and neuralgia. It purifies the blood and cures acne and other skin disorders.

Birch (Betula-Bhoj Patra): Birch extract has been described as astringent, antisepti, softening, curative and circulation-stimulating. They are believed to have curative properties in case of skin diseases. Birch has healing effect on rashes and hair loss. The important constituents include glanonoids, hyproside, tannin, saponins and quercetin. Birch extract has anti-irritant and antiseptic properties in acne, eczema and sunburn. The leaves of plant which have a peculiar, aromatic odour and a bitter taste which secrete a resinous substance with acid properties and contain flavonoids, tannins and essential oils.

Black Pepper Oil: It has cosmetic application, used on skin inflammations and superficial wounds. This oil is obtained from small-grains. The plant, usually is found in hilly areas.

Borage (Pattharchuri): The plant with blue flower have both leaves and stem covered with white bristles. Borge has beneficial effect on heart, kidneys, adrenal glands and the entire digestive system. The herb cures jaundice and increases the milk flow in nursing mothers. Borage juice obtained from the crushed plant and applied direct to the skin cures ringworm. The tropical application of borage extract is described as anti-inflammatory and beneficial for sensitive skin and allergic reactions. Borage contains potassium and calcium, combined with mineral acid. The oil extracted from seed is an effective anti-irritant and has hydrating properties.

Bergamot (Zabeer): An aromatic herb, used to perfume colognes and toilet waters and helps takning. Bergamot oil is considered an antiseptic and bacterial growth inhabitor, good for oily and acne skin and for seborrheilc conditions. Sun exposure after applying pure bergamot oil may cause hyper pigmentation and skin rashes. When the hyper pigmentation seen on the neck area behind the ears.

Carrot Oil: Derived from the carrot root, carrot oil is used since the 16th century for skin diseases due to the cleansing, depurative and draining properties. This carotene-rich emollient has been indicated for acne and skin conditions such as dermatitis, skin irritation, rashes and wrinkles. The root of this plant has nearly 89 per cent water. The extract obtained from the carrot leaves have cleansing properties and healing effect due to its strong antiseptic qualities. The juice contains sugar, a little starch, albumen, volatile oil, vegetable jelly or pectin, saline matter, malic acid and carotin.

Calendula Marigold: Its flowers and leaves are very beneficial for clearing the skin of eczema, spots and grease. It is claimed to be rejuvenating. Calendula extract is an emollient said to have healing, soothing, antiseptic, anti-itching and anti-inflammatory properties. Effectively used in case of oily and delicate skins as well as for curing acne. The extract is obtained from calendula blossom.

Comfrey: A plant with pinkish blue bell-shaped, contains allantoin and is credited with healing, astringent, and emolliengt properties. It is used in case of swelling, bruising, cuts, papules and pustules. The extract is tradionally used topically for soothing and anti-itching treatment (a cold compress for eye injuries), as well as for eczema and wounds. The herb contains from 0.6 to 0.8 per cent of allantoin and a bit of tannin

Celandine: The herb plant is found in hedgerows and wastes. Yellowish hairy leaves shaped like oak leaves and small yellowish flowers. As a wart cure the raw yellow juice should be applied direct to the skin. Some herbalists prescribe an eye lotion made from one part of this infused herb and two parts of water or milk.

Cleavers (Lipatni Ghas): The plant has tiny white flowers and small round fruits. Cleavers are excellent remedy for diseases of the urinary system. An infusion of this herb, used as a lotion, makes a first-rate tonic for the scalp and the skin. It clears dandruff, cures leprosy and skin cancer. The extract is very useful in treating eczema and spots, and is recommended for normal to dry skins.

Clove (laung): An aromatic spice used in skin tonics and stimulating face masks. It is considered as a powerful antiseptic with a strong germicidal effect. Clove oil may cause strong skin irritation when used in high concentration. The clove oil is obtained from the stems and leaves of the plant.

Camomile (Babuna-ka-paudha): Plant with strong botanical properties and feathery gray green leaves, usually found in waster places. The plant has a distinctive smell similar to over-ripe apples. An infusion of leaves and flowers of this plant (fresh or dried) has wide cosmetic and medicinal uses.

Camomile dissolves tumours, heals ulcers, expels worms, banishes tiredness and treats many female disorders. As a cosmetic the herb can be used as a face-wash to clear complexion. Comomile tea is a tonic, digestive and tranquillizing. It is usually sweetened with honey. Camomile oil is considered a antiallargic, healing, cooling, analgesic and antiseptic agent. It has been found exceptionally good for treating burns, skin inflammations and dermatitis.

Cinnamon Oil: Said to have a soothing effect on the skin. It is widely recognised for its tonic and antiseptic properties. It is obtained from the plant's leaves.

Cedarwood Oil: Credited with antiseptic, sedative and astringent properties. This clear oil is valuable for use on various skin eruptions such as relieves itching, cures acne and oily skin, helpful in case of dermatitis eczema and psoriasis.

Dandelion (Kukraundha): The medicinal value of the Dandelion plant with golden-yellow flowers is used to treat all kidney complaints, liver troubles and circulatory disorders. It is widely used for the treatment of arthritis, to disperse acidic deposits from the affected joints. It cures pimples and skin spots.

The dandelion extract has tonic properties, refreshes the skin, corrects pH balance, aids in increasing the respiratory capacity of the skin tissues, beneficial for dry skin and also used in acne preparations. The plant root is used for cosmetic preparations rather than the flower, as juice of the root is more powerful part of the plant. The main constituents of dandelion root are taraxacin (a crystalline bitter substance), taraxacerine (an acid resin), insulin, gluten gum, potash, citric acid, sterols and Vitamin B and C.

Elder (Elder Vriksh): All parts of this herbal plant are used. Its leaves combined with honey is a standard infusion that clears troubled skin. The infused flowers offer a remedy for catarrh, cough and colds. It soothes burns and scalds. A balm of elder flowers keeps crow's feet at bay. The herb is said to have astringent, antiseptic and emollient properties. It is very useful for problem or inflamed skin and the ointment made from the leaves cure bruises, swelling and wounds. They are also ingredient in many cooling ointments. Elder flower extract is used for eye and skin lotions, particularly beneficial for treating dry skin. Elder flower water is used to clear the complexion of freckles and sunburn, and keeps the skin in good condition. Elder flower extract is used for eye and skin lotions, particularly beneficial for treating dry skin. Elder flower water is commonly used to clear the complexion of freckles, sun-burn, and keeps the skin in good condition.

Echin Acea: Both oil and resin derived from the wood or the bark of this aromatic plant have antiseptic and antibacterial properties, helpful in treating skin lesions. It also has anti-itching and soothing properties when used in skin care products and is commonly used in anti-acne preparations.

Elm Bark and Extract: Credited with astringent, healing and soothing properties that could benefit surface skin problems. Extract from elm leaves is usually recommended to wash wounds, bruises and sore eyes.

Eucalyptus: An antiseptic used to fragrance cosmetic preparations. Eucalyptus oil has antiseptic, disinfectant and blood circulation activating properties and is considered one of the most powerful and versatile herbal remedies.

Fennel (Saunf): It is a herb which has a cleansing effect on the skin, especially as a cleanser and detoxifier for oily skin types. When steaming the face, use it in the water. The principal constituents of fennel oil are anethol, fenchone, plus d-pinene, phellandrine, anisic acid and anisic aldehyde.

Fenugreek Extract: An emollient, anti-inflammatory and healing ingredient used in the treatment of irritated skin. The seeds of this herb have been used through the ages for medicinal and culinary purposes.

Garlic (Lahsan): Garlic is included in the same group of plants as the onion. Recognized as an antiseptic and bactericide. The garlic ointment externally applied, reduces hard swelling and for treating skin problem including acne. The active properties of garlic depend on a pungent, volatile, essential oil obtained by distillation. Rich in sulphur, garlic oil helps in clearing skin problems such as eczema and acne.

Geranium Oil: Has botanical properties described as refreshing, anti-irritant, mildly tonic and astringent. It is good for all skin types; particularly benefit oily, inflammatory and acne skins. This oil is used in perfumery and cosmetics.

Henna (Mehandi): An astringent herb with cooling properties. It is used for hair-conditioning. Henna is a colorant that provides a reddish brown shade. It has important constituents, e.g., mucins, phytosterols and napthoquinones. The extract is obtained from the leaves.

Haldi (Turmeric): It helps glow in skin when mixed to a face pack. Adds not only colour, but also prevent flatulence. It prevents inflammation, cures injuries, wounds, used for gonorrhoae (Venereal Disease) and clears eyes relieving pain and redness.

Horse Raddish Extract: Traditionally used against sunburns, superficial and other non extensive burns, and to give the skin clarity and freshness. Its antiseptic and skin clearing properties are linked to its ascorbic acid content. The extract is made primarily from the plant's roots.

Horsetail Extract (Equisetum-ka-paudha): General botanical properties include stimulating, astringent, soothing, healing and softening. Horsetail increases the skin's defense mechanism, regulates the skin due to the plant's rich mineral contents and strengthen connective tissue due to the presence of silicic acid. It works to prevent and counteract wrinkles in the eye area. It is beneficial in both antiaging and relieving acnes.

Houseleek: An herb having healing and astringent properties. Ideal to cure warts and ringworm.

Hyssop Oil (Zufah Yabis): Properties include healing, tonic and stimulating. It is indicated for dermatitis, eczema and wounds. This aromatic plant has long leaves and clusters of light blue flowers. It also regulates blood pressure, clears the chest, calms the nerves, improves digestion and protects the body form infection.

Ivy Extract: Ivy extract has a slimming and anti-cellulite effect due to its ability to prevent water accumulation in the skin tissue. It is considered antibactericidal and soothing, particularly in burn cases. Apparently, ivy also has detergent, anti-parasitic, decongestant and analgesic properties. The leaves are traditionally used to treat various skin eruptions, irritation, dermatitis and skin ulcers.

Jasmine Oil: A highly aromatic oil made from the flowers and used as a perfume. Jasmine may cause allergic reaction (swelling). The oil is credited with moisturizing, soothing and healing properties. It is indicated for dry and sensitive skins, and also for skin with dermatitis.

Lemon: Rich in Vitamin C, it is used in skin tonics and creams. The botanical properties include as acidic, anti-bactericidal and antiseptic. Lemon extract is suggested for treating sunburn, acne problems and oily skin. This extract contains citric acid, Vitamin B and C. Lemon oil is one of the most versatile essential oil, is considered a counter-irritant, antiseptic, depurative and lymphatic stimulant. It is widely used in the perfume and soap industry. Lemongrass oil is the volatile oil distilled from the leaves.

Kaner: Plant with white, yellow and red flowers. Bark of the root cures many skin disorders and purifies the blood. Oil prepared from this plant is useful in cases of scabies and ringworm.

Kalonji (Nigella Sativa): Black seeds resembling onion seeds destroy intestine parasitis. It benefits in cases of gall bladder, calculi, gout, rheumatism and sciatica. Ground in vinegar it helps leucoderma, ringworm, alopecia (patchy baldness) and acne on the face.

Juniper Oil (hapusha): Juniper oil is antiseptic, astringent, cleansing and toning. Also credited with good penetrating capabilities, and is considered helpful in treating acne (oily skin), dermatitis and eczema.

Lavender: It has a pleasant fragrance and used for scenting bath water. Long used as nerve tonic, curing cough, anti-paralytic and used as mouth wash. On external application soothes headaches, reduces inflammation. Properties include antiallergic, anti-inflammatory, antiseptic, antibacterial, anti-spasmodic, balancing, energizing, soothing, healing, tonic and stimulating. Lavender oil works on all types of skins and produces excellent results when used for oily skin as well as in the treatment of acne, burns, dermatitis, eczema and psoriasis.

Lettuce (Chukandar): Rich in minerals, iron and vitamins. It is cooling and excellent for sunburn to redness.

Marigold: The orange marigold is a prolific garden plant. It opens its petals at nine and closes them at four. A disinfectant herb, marigold is used in effective treatment of ulcers and open sores. The flowers may be eaten raw, taken as a standard infusion when applied as a lotion., The plant cures varicose veins and other circulatory troubles. As a lotion, a marigold infusion (petals only) provide the ideal balance of an over-oily skin and all complexions. It has antiseptic, healing and soothing effect and heals sun-burns and skin rashes.

Marjoram (Marwa, Sathra): Described as tonic and anti-fungal. Most popular for botanical applications, Marjoram oil is beneficial for anti-spasmodic, calming and sedative indicating applications for sensitive and irritated skin. Sometimes, it may cause allergic reactions with symptoms being skin redness and itching.

Meadowfoam Oil: A rich emollient. It is widely used in cosmetic formulations because of its dryness and quick penetration into the skin. The extract has strong anti-free radical properties as well as analgesic and topical anti-inflammatory activity. The plant grows abundantly at the edges of the river and ditches.

Mimosa: Used in cosmetics for its believed epidermic tissue regenerating, antiseptic, astringemt, anti-inflammatory, repairing and protecting properties. Used effectively in post-sun preparations, baby skin care creams, and protective creams. It may sometimes produce allergic skin reaction.

Mint (Pudina): Has cooling, tonic, stimulating, antiseptic, digestive and relaxing properties. Mint was traditionally used as an adjunct soothing and anti-itching treatment. This aromatic herb is widely used as a fragrance in beauty products and serves as a cleanser for acne and dermatitis treatment. I cures elephantiasis (swelling in tissues) and varicose veins.

Myrrh: Said to have disinfectant, antiseptic, anti-inflammatory, anti-itching, cicatrizant, tonic, stimulant, sedative and astringent properties. Myrrh extract can be valuable in products designed for acne treatment. Myrrh a traditionally ancient ingredient for perfumes and incense, was used by ancient Egyptian women in facial masks and other cosmetic preparations.

Myrtle: An astringent and antiseptic with strong botanical properties suitable for acne and oily skin.

Neroli Oil: A fragrance, used in skin care preparations to stimulate cell regeneration. It leaves a sedative and soothing effect and most beneficial for sensitive, delicate and all skin types. It is extracted from bitter orange blossom and is one of the most expensive oils, therefore is widely adulterated with the distillation of other citrus blossoms such as sweet orange, lemon and mandarin.

Nettle (Bichchhubooti): The botanical properties include as anti-inflammatory, astringent, bactericidal, healing, mildly deodorant, antioxidant and stimulating. It is effective for treating eczema and sun-burn. Nettle is the botanical with the highest Vitamin E content. Nettle's important constituents include acetylcholine, amino acids, histamine, carotinoids and chlorophyll.

Oak: The botanical properties are described as slightly tonic, strongly astringent, antiseptic, soothing and anti-inflammatory. It reduces inflammation and prevents infection. Oak root is recommended for sensitive skin, protecting it against unwanted reactions such as swelling or redness.

Oat: Oat extract obtained from the seeds of oats has soothing properties on the skin. It helps to enhance emulsion stability, increase viscosity, leave a smooth after feel and provide a source of whole natural vegetable protein. Oatmeal preparations are beneficial for irritated skins resulting from sunburn, psoriasis, or allergic dermatitis. The oatmeal relieves redness and itching. It acts as a soap-free cleanser and provide a gentle base for face masks for delicate, sensitive skin. This mask absorbs oil from the skin's surface and reduce the redness of irritateted, broken-out skin. Oat flour is an abrasive, absorbent, bulking, and viscosity-increasing substance. It is used in a variety of cosmetic preparations including powders, masks, packs, moisturizers, suntan gels, hand and body creams and soaps.

Olive Oil: A carrier oil with excellent lubricity and low odour. Olive leaf extract is astringent and antiseptic, also provides anti-oxidant and vasodilatant properties. It is used in antiaging products.

Orange Flower Oil: Credited with soothing and calming properties when used in skin care preparations. The oil should not be confused with orange flower extract. The flowers from the bitter orange tree yield an essential oil known as neroli.

Palmarosa Oil: The properties attributed to this oil are soothing, moisturizing, antiseptic and cell regeneration. Its used for acne skin and dermatitis codition as well as for dry skin. The oil leaves immediate calming and refreshing action on the skin and is widely used in perfumery and cosmetology.

Pimpernel: This little plant with small oval-shaped leaves, long slender stalks, bearing bright scarlet flower was popular since the ancient Greeks to treat eye diseases, jaundice, dropsy and inflammation. The plant has cosmetic value and is applied as a skin lotion to cure skin pigmentation, removing freckles and blemish and acts as a hair restorer.

Patchouli Oil: Botanical properties of this herb are described as astringent, tonic, sedative, anti-inflammatory and decongestive. Its useful for acne, aged and chapped skin, and skin redness. The oil has strong, sweet and very persistent fragrance.

Peppermint: Credited with refreshing, cooling, bactericidal and anti-irritant properties. It is used as a fragrance, can produced allergic reactions such as skin rashes and irritation, helps relieve skin irritation and itching and reduces skin redness due to inflammation or acne.

Petit Grain Oil: Widely used in pharmacy and perfumery for its therapeutic and tonic effect. It has fresh fragrance and credited with tonic and antiseptic properties.

Pumpkin: Credited with purative properties. Cosmetic applications include use in acne products and as anti-seborrheic.

Quince: Obtained from the dried seeds, its extract is used in cosmetics for dry skin and eye treatment preparations. The seeds are an emollient, emulsifier and thickening agent.

Raspberry: Botanical properties are described as astringent and tonic. The concentrate is added to cosmetics to give them the fruit's fresh smell.

Rose: Rose extract rich in Vitamin C is credited with astringent, tonic and deodorant properties. It is also used as a fragrance. Rose oil has moisturizing and moisture-retention, slightly tonic and soothing properties. It is helpful in case of skin redness or inflammation, when moisturization and regeneration is needed. Rose oil is beneficial to all skin types, particularly mature, dry or sensitive skins. This oil being most expensive essential oils, is largely adulterated with substances like geranium, lemongrass, palmarosa, and terpene alcohols. About 30 roses are required to make one drop of oil. Rose petal extract has mild astrigency and tonic value. Rosewater is credited with cooling, soothing, astringent, and cleansing properties. Rosewater is often mixed with glycerin which provides moisturization and lubricity. Rose oil is one of the major perfumery oils useful as a cellular stimulant and tissue regenerator, especially good to sensitive and aged skin, wrinkles, and general skin care.

Rosemary (Rusemary): A popular garden plant with dark green leaves and distinctive scent. As a medicine, it is valuable tonic for heart and liver and helps reducing high blood pressure. Rosemary is widely used in the treatment of digestive disorders and menstrual pain among women. Used as a lotion, this herb relieves pain in the head and cough, when a spoonful of the herb mixed with honey and melted butter is taken. Rosemary is a fine tonic for the scalp and skin adds luster to the hair and is a useful ingredient in commercial shampoos. It helps to keep the skin free from the wrinkles. Washing the face with rose water keeps the youth alive. The extract have astringent, toning, stimulating, deodorant, antiseptic, reactivating, softening and invigorating properties which helps curing acne, dermatitis and eczema. The constituents of rosemary extract include amino acid, rosemary acid and apigenin.

Sage (Salvia, Sefakuss): An aromatic, sun-loving plant with gray green leaves and mauvish flowers. The herb is used to treat cough, cold, headache, fever, troubles of the liver, bile and the digestive system. When as gargle or mouth wash the herb helps to cure sore throats and gums. The lotion heals ulcers, sores and other skin eruptions such as acne and oily skin. Sage oil is credited with depurative, astringent, invigorating and healing properties.

Sandalwood Oil: Credited with astringent, anti-inflammatory, anti-bacterial, tonic, stimulant, cooling and soothing properties. Beneficial in cases of curing acne and used as astringent for oily skin. The oil may produce rashes on hypersensitive skin, when present in high concentration.

Sesame Oil: It is commonly used as a carrier oil for cosmetic products. It has emollient properties similar to nut and vegetable oil. Sesame oil derived from the seeds is useful is suntan lotions, and reduces 30 per cent of the sun's burning UV rays.

Shahtara (Pitpapda): An herbal plant with fine leaves found in wheat fields with bitter taste and violet flowers. It has been extensively used for disorders arising out of impurities in the blood, like scabies, ringworm besides curing venereal diseases such as Syphilis and gonorrhea.

Sheesham (Red Wood): The oil exuding from this plant is used for many disorders of the skin. It is used as a very efficacious blood purifier curing scabies, ringworm and leucoderma.

Satyanasi (Pela-dhatura): A medicinal plant with yellow flowers and thorny branches. Used as a blood purifier and cures many diseases of the skin. Powder of the seeds use to counter act the itch resulting from venereal diseased, cures scabies and destroys intestinal parasitis.

Sorbitol: Obtained from the leaves. Absorb moisture from the air to prevent skin dryness, leaves the skin feeling smooth and velvety. Used as a replacement for glycerin in emulsions, ointments and various cosmetic creams.

Soapwort Extract (Saboonbooti): It is credited with cleansing and soothing properties. It helps soothing to the skin and relieves itching and inflammation. Soap wart extract is used for treating acne, psoriasis and eczema. The main constituents of this extract made from the roots, leaves and stem include flavonoids and vitamin C, which leave a magic effect on the skin.

Speedwell: The herbal plant with oval-shaped leaves and pale-blue flowers, also known as veronica is prescribed in medicines for treating catarrh, bronchitis, asthma and digestive trouble. Used as a standard infusion internally as well as externally it treats most skin eruptions such as sores, ulcers, pimples, eczema and pruritis. Pure infusion can be applied as an eye lotion to improve the vision in consultation with a Naturopath.

Strawberry: It possesses considerable medical value as well as a remarkable cooling effects on the skin and controls excessive perspiration. Having astringent properties, the herb is useful in dealing with diarrhea, menstruation disorders threatened abortion, risk of haemorrhage and the digestive system. Strawberry juice can be used to treat more serious skin ailments. It contains maximum iron contents and cures anemia. It helps curing more serious skin ailments such as eczema, pruritis and sunburned skins.

Thyme (Ban Ajwain): The herb grows wild on dry banks and heaths, has woody stems and flattish round leaves and heavily scented flowers. Thyme have cleansing properties and its poultice made from leaves combat inflammation and infection. Thyme is digestive used as a liver tonic and cures a wide range of psychological disorders, headaches, hysteria, halitosis and various female ailments. Thyme oil obtained from branches and flowers is considered a powerful product having botanical properties such as antiseptic, tonic, antibacterial, deodorizing, fungicidal and circulation stimulating. The oil is obtained from the herb's branches and flowers.

Tamarind (Imli): Credited with astringent, antiseptic and strong immuno-stimulating properties. Constituents of this plant include citric, tartaric and malic acids, potassium bitartrate, polysaccharides, proteins and lipids. This botanical is recommended for protecting the skin against environmentally induced damage, stimulating skin repair and for skin with low immuno defenses.

Tea Tree Oil: A natural preservative with antiseptic, germicidal and expectorant properties. The oil cures skin disorders and infections of all type of skins. It helps to fight against seborrhea, psoriasis, scaling and redness of skin, eczema, itching and dermatitis.

Turmeric: Credited to healing, tonic, mildly stimulating, anti-inflammatory and blood-purifying properties. This herb is useful for a variety of curative purposes including the treatment of acne, eczema, skin infections, ulcers, burns and rashes.

Vervain: The plant having green-gray leaves and small hooded mauve flowers has properties to cure nervous disorders, epilepsy, asthma, relieves disorders of the liver, heart and spleen. It relieves mental strain and helps cure infectious diseased, used as gargle or mouth-wash for sore throats and gums and as an eye lotion. It is also recommended for curing inflammation and diseases of skin.

Walnut: The extract obtained from leaves and bark of the plant is traditionally used topically soothing and anti-itching, as well as against sunburns and other superficial burns. It can be used in case of acne and other skin diseases because of its fungi static and astringent properties.

Witch Haze: Traditionally used in topical treatment of burns, sunburns, skin irritation, insect bites and bruises. It is credited with anti-inflammatory, wound-healing, anti-itching, softening and emollient properties.

Yarrow (Sahastrapani, Gandana): Having grayish, feathery, leaves and small daisy-like flowers, yarrow has been used since antiquity for headaches, fevers (influenza), diarrhoea paltipations and excessive menstruation. The extract have astringent, antiseptic, anti-inflammatory, healing and calming properties. The important constituents include flavonoid, amino acids, sugars and phytosterols. It is beneficial for oily and acne skins.

Cactus Extract: An emulsifier for creams and lotions described as good for sunburns and other minor burns, insect bites, skin irritations, swelling and inflammations. It is used for face masks.

Cosmetic Use of Herbs

For those in search of beauty and lost youth, herbs have always held a special fascination, and one that our modern cosmetic industry have exploited. For this reason the cosmetic use of herbs is a subject to those intent on finding beauty. To maintain youth or beauty, people spend a lot, some on surgeons to stitch up double chins or de-bag eyes, others on expensive creams to banish acne and wrinkles. And despite all this, everybody ages and nothing can do stop it. Where certain herbs can help, perhaps, is in improving the faces we were born with and, where possible, delaying the more obvious marks of ageing. In other words, herbs will not create youth a beauty, but will enable us to make the most of what we have of either. An early experimenter in the field of herbal cosmetics was the Greek physician Galen who invented cold cream. He hit upon the idea of melting together white wax and oil of roses in a particular ratio; and then stirring into this mixture a cupful of water laced with spirit vinegar. Since Galen's time the oil of roses has been replaced by almond oil or even liquid paraffin, although the best substitute is sunflower oil particularly rich in vitamin A and Vitamin D.

Making Your Own Cosmetics

Make good use of all kinds of everyday items like fruit, vegetables, nuts, cereals in nurturing their beauty. Even in most beauty conscious there is a definite tendency towards natural therapies. The kitchen larder is a storehouse of beauty aids. You just have to follow a few recipes, pick the ingredients, mix them in a required ratio and you will soon have a beauty lotion or cream in hand. These home-made herbal preparations help enhance beauty of the skin and complexion and delay ageing without causing harm. Taking care of your skin is a must in order to remain young. During youth the skin is elastic and smooth but as one grows older, the skin loses its elasticity, natural oils and water content. In days gone by, there were hardly any cosmetics available in the market and rural areas, and home made preparations were used for skin care. Since ancient times vegetable oils, refined animal fats and cream of milk have been used for the care of the skin and beauty. A number of costly modern creams available in the market today are still based on refined animal fat. These help in keeping the skin smooth.

Making your own creams, lotions is easy. By learning to make your own cosmetics, you cosmetics, you have at your finger-tips not only more luxurious products than you could afford to buy but also those especially suitable for your skin. Most of the recipes mentioned in this book have been tested and are extremely easy to make. Creams and emulsions are all basically a mixture of water and oily substances, waxes and fragrances in varying proportions. A slight change in proportion change the character of the preparation. Be careful when measuring the ingredients. When measuring the quantity the following rough equivalents should be kept in mind:

60 drops = 1 teaspoon (tps) = 5 ml

3 teaspoons = 1 tablespoon (tbs) =15 ml

2 tablespoon = 1/8 cup or 16 tablespoons = 1 cup

1000 ml = 1 litre = 1. 759 pints (or 1 pint = 0.568 litre)

15. 4 grains = 1 gm

16 ozs = 0. 453 kilograms

1 kg = 2. 20 lbs

Some Dos and Don'ts: The following dos and don'ts should be kept in mind when making a herbal preparation at home:

- Do not expose oils and waxes to direct heat as these can burn and an intense heat can change the properties of the preparation.
- When heating oils and waxes, put them in separate enamel bowls, placed in a large pan filled with hot water (not boiling) and continue stirring with either a wooden spoon or a glass rod or a slow speed electric heater. While stirring, add water to the wax or the oils if it is too thick.
- Add perfume or colouring matter when the preparation is ready and in case of a cream, mix it when it cools and thickens. In case your skin is sensitive or allergy-prone, it is advised to omit perfume.
- Ensure that the contents of the preparation are properly mixed otherwise preparation may turn gritty. Make sure to continue stirring or beating until the cream is cool. If the preparation does not gel, melt it again and repeat the process. You may add a few drops of oleic acid to bind together any cream or lotion.
- The herbal ingredients used in preparing the cosmetics may be easily available with leading 'pansari' shops or a herbal store or dispensing chemists.
- Bees wax, emulsifying wax and cocoa butter can be available with a dispensing chemist. Lanolin is readily available with the chemists. These are usually of two types- anhydrous and hydrous. Anhydrous lanolin is commonly used because it has less water contents. In case, anhydrous lanolin is not readily available, you may procure hydrous lanolin, which has in itself a fairly large water contents. The preparations with anhydrous lanolin will be much more richer and greasier. Oils, herbs, lentils, fuller's earths, camphor, etc. can be purchased from a 'pansare' shop or a good herbalist.

- Home-made herbal cosmetic preparations have a short life, which can be lengthened by storing them in a refrigerator. It is suggested to make a small quantity of the recipe and use them lavishly while still fresh. Keep a small jar in the bathroom and the rest in the refrigerator. Nepagin M is an effective preservative. When heating the contents, add a few drops of Nepagin M. Stir constantly until the oily globules disperse. This will enhance the shelf life of preparation.

Fruits, Vegetables and Natural Substances Used in Ayurveda. Here is a brief description of some of the very useful ingredients required in making Ayurvedic preparations for health and beauty:

Amla (Emblice Myrobalan): Cheapest source of vitamin C which is not destroyed by boiling or other process. A good substance for hair washing and helps in case of falling and premature graying of hair. It rejuvenates the body.

Anar (Pomegranate): A delicious juicy fruit with many medicinal properties, It is cooling and allays uncontrollable thirst in diarrhea, digestive. Flowers of the plant are an ingredient for miscarriage. The rind of fruit is an astringent and have a tonic effect on the tissues. Bark of root of the plant is used in case of intestinal worms.

Alcohol: It has antiseptic, preserving and grease cutting properties. Used mainly in stimulating stringent and as a solvent for essential oils. Vodka is a common substitute for alcohol.

Arand Kharbuza: Also called as golden tree of life which acts as a digestive agent because of arbge amounts of pepsin. It is used to reduce inflammation of live and spleen. The sap of tree cures ringworm and intestinal parasites.

Alum: A fine white or yellow powder with astringent properties, also knows as 'fitkari'. It is used in lotions and as dry shampoo to remove sweat and dirt.

Apple: A naturally acid fruit good for the skin. Apple cider restores the acid mantle to the skin. Can be used as skin tonic.

Apricot (Khubani): Rich in Vitamin A. Use the pulp in face masks. Apricot oil is very rich in poly-unsaturated oil, so it is used in nourishing creams.

Banana: Nourishing and used in masks.

Beeswax: Also known as 'madhu-mom'. It is an ester wax with a high melting point. Ideal for face creams. An emulsifier when mixed with borax. It takes eight parts of honey to produce one part of beeswax. It is one of the oldest raw ingredients used in cosmetic preparations, Beeswax is used as part of the wax composition of solid and paste products such as creams, lipstick and pomades. Beeswax is credited with anti-inflammatory, anti-allergic, anti-oxidant, anti-bactericidal, germicidal, skin softening and elasticity enhancing properties. It rarely cause sensitivity, and allergy reaction. Bleached beeswax is white whereas unbleached beeswax is yellow.

Beer: Used to wash the face and as a hair setting lotion. It prevents skin rashes.

Barley: It has nutritional value and is rich in iron and vitamin B. It cools the body, strengthens the nerves, and is excellent tonic food during convalescence.

Basil (Tulsi): Has blood purifying qualities. It is used for ringworm, scabies, leucoderma and even leprosy.

Benzoin: A fragrant essential oil with bactericidal, anti-irritation and anti-itching properties. It is considered a good ingredient for reducing skin redness and is also a preservative of fats. While its primary constituent is benzoic acid, it also contains vanillin and an oily aromatic liquid. Also known as 'lohban'.

Borax (Suhaga): It has mild detergent and anti-septic properties. Used as emulsifier in conjunction with bees-wax. It cures the patient of ringworm.

Bade (Banyan Tree): It is also known as Bodhi tree. It has many medicine properties to prepare formulations for spermatorrhae, premature ejaculation etc. Sap of its leaves is a specific for kibes and corns.

Bakain (Lilac): A tree resembling neem. The leaves have blood purifying properties; recommended for scabies, ringworm, leprosy, leucaderma and to reduce inflammation.

Calamine Lotion: An alkaline lotion used to soothe irritated skin. It contains lime water, glycerin, zinc oxide and calamine.

Camphor: A white crystalline substance used as an anti-septic. It is healing and soothing when used on spot. It is used either camphor cake or camphor spirit. Camphor oil is stimulating.

Castor Oil (Arandi Ka Tel): A rich oil used in hair products. Leaves of the tree smeared with sesame oil and applied to inflammations tend to relieve them. It has many medicine used also.

Carrot Juice (Gajar Ka Ras): Rich in vitamin A, B and C. Used in nourishing eye creams. Carrot oil have cleansing, depurative and draining properties and cures acne, dermatitis, wrinkles and skin irritation.

Cocoa Butter: Solidified waxy oil from the roasted cocoa beans, used as lubricant in massage creams. It is good for dry skins.

Corn Oil (Gram Seed Oil): A heavy vegetable oil which can be used in body and face creams.

Coconut Oil: Used as a cream base. A raw material in soaps, ointments, massage creams and in sunscreen formulations. It may be irritating to the skin and cause skin rashes.

Caraway Oil (Carum Carvi): A carrier oil having ability to remove bruises, and believed to have tissue regenerating properties. It is beneficial for acne (oily) skin.

Citric Oils: Refers to one or a combination of oil from citrus fruits such as orange oil, lemon oil, grapefruit oil and the like.

Corn Oil: Used as a carrier oil. This vegetable oil has average emollient properties. It is widely used in cosmetic formulations.

Cotton Seed Oil: The oil is used in the manufacture of soaps, creams and baby creams. It is known to cause allergies and be mildly irritating. Expressed from various species of cotton.

Cucumber: It is slightly astringent, cool and refreshing, and used in lotions, creams and masks.

Cucumber extract is credited with moisture-binding, moisture-regulating, soothing, tightening, anti-itching, refreshing, softening, healing and anti-inflammatory properties. It contains amino acids and organic acids that are claimed to strengthen the skin's acid mantle. The extract can be used in after shave preparations, eye treatment products and treatment for oily skin. It is also effective in emulsions as a tightening agent for stressed skin and in suntar preparations.

Fuller's Earth (Multani Mitti): An absorbent clay, rich in minerals. Used in face masks for thickening and cleansing, drawing and stimulating. Also used as dry shampoo. A paste on the skin cures prickly heat.

Eggs: The most useful aid to beauty. The yolk is nourishing and the white is drying and tightening. Used in masks and as a hair conditioner. Egg protein creates a film, thereby acting as a moisture-retention agent allowing the skin to build up a supply of water. The moisturizing process tightens and softens the skin only temporarily as the skin cannot utilize the protein contained in a egg. It may cause skin rashes and other disorders in those with an allergy to eggs. Egg lecithin is recommended for sensitive skins. The egg oil extracted form the egg yolk is recommended for sensitive skins. The egg yolk extract is a protein with emulsifying capabilities, contains lecithin sterols and Vitamin A.

Emulsifying Wax: Extremely useful for stabilizing creams. Made from ceto stearyl alcohol and sodium lauryl sulphate. It is an emulsifier and thickening agent used to give body to a formulation. Unlike some waxes including beeswax, this is not a true wax. It is a chemical mixture of emulsifiers and fatty alcohols that permit the formulation of stable creams.

Glycerin: Attracts and holds moisture. Used in face creams and lotions. Glycerin is used in moisturizers due to its water-binding capabilities that absorb water from the air. Glycerin helps the skin retain moisture. Glycerin also improves the spreading qualities of creams and lotions. It is clear syrupy liquid made by chemically combining water and fat that is usually derived from vegetable oil.

Gelatine: A rich source of protein. used for hair conditioning or diluted as a setting lotion and nail hardening cream.

Glucose: Has moisture-binding properties and provides the skin with a soothing effect. It is a sugar that is generally obtained by the hydrolysis of starch.

Grapes: Slightly acid and good for cleansing and bleaching. It is described as tonic, with anti-inflammatory and decongestant properties. It may act as an antioxidant. Grapes are beneficial in anti-aging, after-sun and other sun care products. Grape seed oil has moisturizing and nourishing properties due to its high linoleic acid content.

Groundnut Oil: A vegetable oil used in face creams and body lotions. Also known as peanut oil.

Gum Resin: Used as a tightening, fixing and stabilizing agent in the cream. It can be dissolved in water.

Honey: Healing, nourishing and softening. It is used in masks, cream and lotions. A perfect food if taken with milk or lime water. It is helpful incases of paralysis and cures suppurating (pussy) wounds and improve eye sight.

Hydrogen Peroxide: A bleaching and oxidizing agent, detergent and antiseptic. A skin bleacher in cosmetics. If used undiluted, it can cause burns of the skin and mucous membranes.

Hydrolyzed Milk Protein: Forms a film on the skin's surface that allows the skin to retain moisture.

Kaolin (China Clay): Often-used in powders and masks, It is appropriate absorber of the oil and sweat secreted by the skin.

Lanolin: A thick tacky fat, widely used in skin foods for its moisturizing and softening effects. Lanolin is an emollient with moisturizing properties and an emulsifier with high water absorption capabilities.

Linseed Oil: Botanical properties are listed as emollient, anti-inflammatory, and healing. Derived from the flax plant seed obtained by expression with liyyle or no heat.

Lovage Oil: A scribed botanical properties such as cleansing, depurative, and draining make lovage oil appropriate for use on oily skin.

Lecithin Powder: A complex, highly nutritious soft yellow powder found in egg yolk and soybeans. It is an natural emollient, emulsifier, antioxidant, and spearing agent that attracts water and acts as a moisturizer.

Neem (Margosa Tree): Bitter leaves used as an antiseptic. Neem leaves when ground in paste and applied relieve prickly heat, remove pus from wounds, clean boils on the skin. All parts of the tree are endowed with the quality of purifying blood.

Mint (Pudina): Extensively used in cooking, has great digestive properties. It cures elephantiasis and varicose veins. Beneficial in case of urtiearia.

Milk: Used for softening, nourishing and cleaning the skin. Milk protein gives a smooth feel to the skin.

Milk protein, primarily is well absorbed by the skin and gives it gloss and fine touch by forming a soft film.

Oatmeal (Jai Ka Atta): A cleansing and soothing meal. Use it for washing with, or in masks. Finelly ground oatmeal is found in any grocer's shop.

Oak: Oak leaves in the bath are deodorant and relaxing. They soothe inflammation.

Onion: An antiseptic. Wash your face with onion juice to prevent blemishes and mix it with honey to make an anti-wrinkle cream. Juice of onion taken in conjunction with honey and eggs, it is an excellent tonic with aphrodisiac qualities. An excellent preparation against cholera and diarrholea if steeped in vinegar.

Orange: Contains Vitamin C. The juice is used in skin tonics and masks. Dry and grind some orange peel and use it in masks and facial scrubs. Also used in toothpowders.

Olive Oil: A poly-unsaturated vegetable oil used in nourishing creams. Olive oil is a carrier oil with excellent lubricity, pale colour, and low odour. Olive oil is considered an especially good carrier for essential oils.

Papaya: It is also called paw-paw. Softening and cleansing. The enzymes in the fruit have a deep cleansing effect by breaking down the dead cells of the skin. It contains calcium, iron, phosphorus and magnesium salt.

Peach: Moisturizing, nourishing and delicious smelling. Use the mashed pulp on dry, rough skin in skin tonics and masks.

Petroleum Jelly: A lubricating jelly often used in cleansing creams, and hand and nail creams.

Paraffin: Used in cosmetics as a beeswax substitute. Paraffin is a solid mixture of hydrocarbons obtained from petroleum. Presence of impurities in paraffin may result in irritation, eczema and other skin problems.

Panwar (Mihndi): A herb growing in wastelands. Has seeds like kidney beans. Ground seed applied to skin cures ringworm, leucoderma and blemishes.

Palmitic Acid: Obtained from palm oil, one of the skin's major fatty acids produced by the sebaceous glands. In cosmetic preparations, it is used as a formula texturizer.

Peanut Oil: Utilized as a skin softener, emulsifier and emollient. It is used as a substitute for expensive oils such as almond and olive in cosmetic creams. Peanut oil has a higher Vitamin A, Vitamin E and nicotinic acid content than other nut oils.

Potatoes: Have cleansing and drawing properties. Clears the skin. Use thin raw potato slices for eyepads to remove puffiness of eyes.

Resin: Used to give gloss, flow, adhesion and water resistance to cosmetics. This is a brittle substance, usually translucent or transparent, that can be either derived naturally or synthetically obtained.

Retinol: Considered a skin revitalize, retinal is reported to enhance skin radiance and treat conditions associated with ageing such as wrinkles, fine lines, acne and papules.

Safflower Oil: A rich poly-unsaturated oil suitable for all nourishing cosmetics. A carrier oil considered hydrating to the skin, is obtained from the seeds and have astringent, anti-inflammatory and soothing properties especially for sensitive skin and areas with burns.

St. John's Wort Oil (Basant): Considered anti-inflammatory. It is beneficial for sensitive and/or rough, chapped skin as well as skins suffering from acne, irritation and inflammatory circulation.

Sodium Chloride (Salt): Used as a preservative, astringent and antiseptic to treat inflame lesions. Sodium sisqui is a powdery substance which is a water softener and is used in bath salts. Salt is used with equal parts of bicarbonate of soda as an excellent tooth powder. Also used as an abrasive body rub to tone the skin and improve circulation.

Sodium Bicarbonate (Baking Soda): An inorganic salt used as a buffering agent and a pH adjuster. Used in skin smoothing powders and also serves as a neutralizer.

Sodium Bisulphate: An organic salt used as an buffering agent and a pH adjuster in cosmetic creams.

Sarson (Mustard): A well-known oil seed. The seeds of the plant used for extracting oil used for massage, as cooking medium and also as hair oil.

Stearic Acid: A natural fatty acid. It is crystalline, white, waxy substance, which gives pearliness to creams, hand and body lotions.

Sugar: An abrasive face scrub. Lather the face with soap, then add a handful of sugar and scrub, rinse off and apply lemon juice. This thoroughly cleanses and stimulates the skin.

Sulphur: A yellow powder used in acne preparations. It helps slow down the activity of the oil producing glands. Some people are allergic to it, so before using it on your face, give yourself a skin test behind the ear.

Tea: Contains tannin which has a soothing and healing effect. It absorbs ultra-violet light and is used in sun creams to help prevent burning. Tea bags are marvellously soothing ready made eye pads.

Soybean Oil: Used as a smoothing ingredient. It has high content of phosphate ides such as lecithin, sterols and Vitamins (A, E and K). Soyabean oil is not irritating.

Spermaceti: A waxy substance used in the manufacture of cosmetics, to thicken the products and give them shine. Spermaceti is non-toxic and non-irritating.

Tamanu Oil: Used for the improvement of cell regeneration. It can be found in products used to protect the skin against sun exposure, as well as ant aging formulations to cure wrinkles.

Tomato: A slightly acidic vegetable containing potassium and Vitamin C. Use it on blackheads, open pores and greasy skin.

Turtle Oil: Vitamin enriched oil. Often used in rich nourishing creams. It but smells bad.

Vinegar: Acidic. Use diluted eight parts water to one part vinegar. Improves and softens the skin.

Vetiver Oil (Khus-Khus): Produced from the roots of a fragrant grass. Considered stimulant and tonic, and used in perfumery as well as in cosmetics.

Vervain Oil: Has been credited with astringent and antispasmodic properties.

Vitamins: Valuable for skin and hair. Vitamin A can pass through the skin and is useful for dry skin and acne. Also have soothing properties. Vitamin B promotes health of skin and hair. Vitamin C promotes healing of acne. Vitamin D can be absorbed through skin and has a healing effect on the skin. Vitamin E is said to have healing properties. Vitamin F counteracts dry, chapped skin. Greatly used in face and hand creams, and in hair treatments to counteract brittle hair.

Wheatgerm Oil: Made from twigs of hamamelis or alder bush. Widely used in skin tonics for its astringent properties. Traditionally used in topical treatment of burns, sun-burns, skin irritation, insect bites and bruises. It is credited with anti-inflammatory and wound healing properties. It is used for its ant-itching, softening and emollient properties.

Yoghurt: A liquor made from milk. It contains enzymes. Used as a base for cleansing and cleaning face masks.

9

Nature Cure for Skin Disease

Disorder	*Symptoms*	*Causes*	*Cure*
Acne vulgaris	Blackheads and spots	Sebaceous ducts are chocked with dirt	Clean the skin thoroughly. Ground together the barks of Oris Tree (Irsa), Neem and Turmeric in water. Rub on the affected skin.
Boils and Pustules	Red, swelling, itching, forms round a hair	Bacterial infection	Black cumin (kali jeeri) ground in water and apply paste on the boils.
Birthmarks	Dark brown patches to fleshy bumps. Small moles	Scratching of pimples, after effect of small pox	Massage with carbon snow. Peeling treatment. Skin grafting a surgeon.
Cracked skin	Chapped skin	Defective functioning of sebaceous glands	Smear ghee or mustard oil over the affected skin or apply milk cream at night.
Corns	Painful hardening and thickening of skin of the feet	Chaffing shoes	Cut it off with a sharp knife or razor and apply the sap of the papaya tree over it. It should be covered with a cut lemon and bandaged.

Disorder	*Symptoms*	*Causes*	*Cure*
Crow's Feet	Lines and wrinkles on face. Skin hangs in folds and wrinkles appear around eyes	Ageing	Apply sesame or coconut oil over the face and neck before sleep. The anger and irritation add to the lines of age on the face. Douche with warm and then cold water alternatively. Avoid rubbing the skin
Dermatitis	Itchy skin, Red patches and flaking of skin	Sensitive Skin. Effect of cosmetics	Application of moist warm compresses of potassium permanganate solution.
Eczema	Inflammation with watery discharge without itching	Digestive derangements	Apply paste of Babchi mixed with mustard oil or leaves of Mahua (Indian Butter Tree) smeared with sesame oil should be applied.
Freckles	Brownish spots	Precipitation of pigments or exposure to sun	Ground yellow mustard in milk and apply at night. Wash face thoroughly in the morning OR make a paste of turmeric and sesame seeds (in equal quantity) and apply.

Disorder	*Symptoms*	*Causes*	*Cure*
Genital scabies	Lesions on genitals. Intense nocturnal	Scratching leaves small shallow ulcer and crusting	Identify source of allergic reaction.
Herps	Blisters appear on skin, mostly on genitals. Other affected areas include thighs and buttocks	Infection. In case of genital herbs, due to having sex with someone who has herpes	Apply anti-viral cream/ lotion; use condoms during sex. Apply warm salt-water bath. Worry, depression lack of sleep makes condition worst.
Kibes	Cracking of heels; some-times painful condition	Wearing shoes without socks	Fill the crack with the sap of Banyan tree. Apply prepared ointment by mixing sesame oil, finely ground resin and beeswax to be cooked for few minutes.
Leucoderma	White patches on the skin	Loss of pigmentation of the skin	Steep in water equal quantity of Babchi and Tamarind seeds for 3-4 days. Grind and apply on affected skin.
Leprosy	Formation of massive nodules	Nerves are destroyed.	Massage with the sap of the neem tree.

Disorder	*Symptoms*	*Causes*	*Cure*
Prickly Heat	Profuse sweating and red pustules of the size of mustard grains on body with intense itch on chest, back and abdomen	Excessive heat and sun exposure	Smear pack of Multani Mitti dissolved in water over affected parts. Apply green henna leaves ground in water. Alternatively, white sandal or tender leaves of Neem ground in water also help.
Psoriasis (Eka Kushta)	Raised, rough, reddened areas with silvery scale on the Body	Impurities in the blood associated with emotional factors	Guggulu Tiktaka Ghrita is given internally to improve digestion and remove impurities from the blood. Spicy food, curds and salt should be avoided. May use a little rock salt. Neem tree leaves (grinded) applied on the area will be helpful.
Pigmentation of skin	Discoloration of skin, scarring and blemishes	Exposure to sun. Allergy to perfume	
Ring Worm	Pustules or sores on the skin, usually between legs or scrotum, on neck, the back and buttocks	Inflammatory infection	Apply juice of marigold (genda) or tulsi leaves.

Disorder	*Symptoms*	*Causes*	*Cure*
Scabies	Irritation, itch of skin	Tiny organism	Juice of lemon and Jasmine mixed; applied on the affected area.
Small Pox scars	Permanent marks on face	Fever	Sprinkle face with hot and cold water alternatively to activate blood circulation. Apply coconut oil and pat lightly for five minutes. The scars may not vanish totally but would be less prominent.
Sun burn	Dryness of skin, scarring and wrinkles.	Adverse effect of sun	Apply face mask of a mixture of bleaching powder and hydrogen peroxide. Apply suntan lotion.
Urticaria (Nettle rash)	Rashes (raised red and white patches) appear on whole body with swear itching	Digestive disorders and allergic reaction	Equal quantity of Alum and Red Ochra (Geru) should be ground together and the powder rubbed on the weals. In case of severe itching, mix 3 parts rose water and 2 parts vinegar and apply on the affected area. Avoid exposure to hot and cold water.

Disorder	*Symptoms*	*Causes*	*Cure*
Whitlow	A small, painful abcess forms at the base of nail or pulp of finger with intense pain	Due to inflammation of deep seated tissues in the finger	One part Isphagula should be steeped in four part of Vinegar and apply to the spot, the inflammation is likely to resolve in 2-3 days. Once the pus has been ejected, neem should be made into a poultice and bound over the affected site.
Warts	Brownish epidermal growths. Swelling	Caused by Virus	Apply peeling agent daily. Apply solicyclic acid. Freezing with liquid nitrogen or carbon snow.

Nature Cure for Hair Disorders

Disorder	*Symptoms*	*Causes*	*Cure*
Hair loss	Temporary or permanent falling of hair	Mental tension, stress, use of substandard cosmetics, over dry or greasy hair etc.	Should take a vigorous massage of the scalp. If new hairs are not replaced when the patient gets total baldness. The hair should be combed with the fingers and dried through massage
Alopecia	Patchy round baldness	Usually occur in old age, sometimes premature baldness even at young age due to worry, mental tension & over work	Daily massage for 15 to 30 minutes. Apply carbonic snow (dry ice) which gives an alternate cold and hot feeling. Dissolve few grains of potassium permanganate in water (or three cloves of garlic together with a pinch of collyrium) and apply on bald patches. If there is any irritation, smear butter over the patch.

Dandruff (Pityriasis)	Uppermost layer of scalp continuously cast off and shedding scales	Excessive secretion of the sebaceous glands	Massage scalp with pure apple juice (one part) mixed to warm water (three parts) three times a week. Rosemary infusion (5 tablespoon) and borax lotion (a pinch) cure dandruff when massaged into the scalp daily. Dab with diluted cosmetic vinegar into the scalp, parting the hair at bed time.
Dullness of Hair	Dry Hair	Washing hair with hard water. Dietory deficiency	Apply cold beer over head. Mix olive oil with 2 egg and use as hair mask.
Eczema	Itchy Scalp	Effect of chlorine, salt and chemicals in hair	Use medicated shampoo. Use mild vinegar rinse before shampoo. Apply egg shampoo mixed with orange juice.
Flackiness	Itchy scalp. White flacks on hair	Not rinsing hair thoroughly after shampoo	Use extra sunflower oil in your daily diet. Avoid being under stress during periods.

Thinning of hair	Hair is sparsely spaced	Due to heredity, illness and excessive teasing or brushing	Gently brushing or combing the hair. Weekly massage with a warm oil. Avoid use of hair spray and sleep with the rollers on.
Hair with split ends	Hair with twin face	Brushing wet hair or excessive use of hair dryer	Apply hair conditioner. Avoid use of hair dryer and hot rollers. Massage into the scalp with olive oil, steam and then shampoo the hair.
Premature Grey Hair	Worry and shock. Washing hair with too hot water. Chronic cold and sinusitis	Sudden shock, illness, colouring, hair perming, bleaching or use of sub-standard cosmetics	Chemical darkening agents should be avoided. Open air, exercise, massage of scalp, dietary regimen, ingestion of raw vegetables are recommended.
Lice Infestation	Lices accumulates in scalp & hair	Insanitary condition of the hair	Wash the hair with juice of lemon mixed with luke warm water. Take a diet of fruits and vegetables for some weeks.

Nature Cure for the Genito-Urinary and Reproduction Organs

Kidney Disorder

Disorder	Symptoms	Causes	Cure
Renal Colic	Pain in the kidneys	Inflammation	Two parts Black cumin seeds, one part ajwain and a pinch of black salt, ground together and mix with a little vinegar taken in a little quantity every hour till relief obtained. Alternatively, as for local applications, two egg yolks should be beaten in a copper vessel. Add to it turmeric and a little water. It should be warmed and applied as a poultice to the region of kidney.

Dysuria	Scanty discharge, pain while urinating, pain in the penis (in men) and ovaries (in women), blood while urinating, heaviness in kidneys and urge for frequent urination	Cystitis, inflammation of the bladder and urethra, venereal disease like gonorrhoea and enlargement of the prostate gland within the pelvis. Hyperacidity (excessive amount of acid present in urine)	Desist from eating beans and pulses. Avoid eating green vegetable e.g. spinach, tomatoes and ladyfinger. Constipation should be avoided. Most important drug used for this condition is 'shilajita' followed by the compounded preparations 'chandraprabha vati'.
Stones	Severe pains in kidneys and bladder	Infection	Drink every morning and evening juice of Radish mixed with pearl ash (jawakhar) for few days to break up the stones and expelled with urine.
Scalding Urine	Burning sensation during urination	Hyperacidity or malfunctioning of kidneys	Boil 250 gms milk with an equal quantity of water and drink. Alternatively, grind 50 gms of rattanjot booti with 5 grains of pepper in water. Strain and drink it after sweetening it with sugar candy.

Polyuria	Excess of urine (amount increases in winter and decreases in summer)	Excessive intake of liquids or failure of sweat glands to function	Eat a confection from black sesame seeds; can be prepared by mixing 4 parts seeds, 2 parts ajwain and 6 parts of jaggery taken twice daily in the morning and evening. Alternatively, the kernel of tamarind seeds and leaves of horse radish should be ground together in water and apply luke warm to the pelvic region.
Haematuria	Presence of blood in urine. Smoky or brownish colour urine	Stone in kidneys scratched urethera	Mix a pinch of turmeric (haldi) in 100 gms dried amla. Crush and steep overnight in water. The water should be given to the patient in the morning.

Urinary calculi	Pain	Formation of stone in kidney or ureter	Consult doctor for treatment.
Syphilis (V.D.)	Contagious disease, shows signs of decay resembling those caused by leprosy	Acquired by sexual intercourse with a person suffering from disease	Ground in water 20gm of Hirankhuri booti (corchorus fascicularis) and five grains of pepper. Strain and take for two three weeks (consult a doctor also).
Gonorrhoea (VD)	Inflammation affecting the mucous membrane of the urethra in male and the vagina in the female. It spreads to other parts of body. Intense irritation of the urethra, pain on passing urine with which a yellow viscid discharge comes out	Through sexual contact with partner suffering from this dreaded disease	Seek doctor's advice. Hip bath in hot water is useful. The urethra should be flushed with a solution of potassium permanganate (1:3,000) with the help of a syringe, which may be kept in the urethra for five minutes.

Amenorrhoea	Scanty discharge of menstrual blood or absence of menses flow due to faulty functioning of ovaries	Due to conditions e.g. anaemia, grief resulting stoppage of menses for months due to slow or imperfect development of the ovaries or womb	Do not over-strain yourself mentally or physically. Hot and cold hip baths and sunbathing will be helpful.
Displacement of uterus	Backache or head ache, heaviness in the bowels. Patient feels that something is sticking to uterus	The downwards displacement of uterus is known as prolapse and in this condition the uterus slips between rectum and bladder.	The best way to deal with the problem is naturopathic way e.g. fasting, improvement in diet and exercises to tone up the muscle supporting the uterus.
Lucorrhoea	White or pale watery discharge from the uterus. The discharge may be thick consisting pus.	Infection or chronic inflammation of the womb following child-bearing and a venereal disease	Exercise the body by running, playing and household work. Take every morning a dose of dried and powdered bark of the mulsari (Minusops Elengi) tree mixed to an equal quantity of brown sugar with water. Avoid fried, spicy food and pickles. Late nights and sexual intercourse are taboo during the course of disease.

Menorrhagia	Excessive bleeding during mestruation	Faulty functioning of ovaries.	Hot and cold hip bath.
Metrorrhagia	Excessive bleeding from onset of puberty	-do-	-do-
Nocturnal Emission	Seminal discharge during sleep	Mental tension. Sexy TV programmes/adult movies.	Hot and Cold hip bath.
Apprehension of miscarriage	Pain or the slightest bleeding	Excess burden or mental tension by the expectant mothers	The foot of the bed should be kept raised a couple of inches for a few hours in the day when the patient is on bed rest. A wet pack should be placed on the pubes for an hour in the morning and evening. The process should be repeated on the dates the pregnant woman would have had her period. After the third month the apprehension of a miscarriage will recede.

Threatened Abortion	Spotting (a drop or two of blood oozing out of uterus)	Heavy physical or mental work	Take amla wrapped in silver foil daily during pregnancy or, a confection of petals of white rose.
Phospaturia	A whitish liquid follows urination	Sexual weakness or disorder	Defective digestion can give rise to emission of phosphates. Tone up the digestive processes the naturopathic way.
Vaginitis	Blood stained discharge	local infection, burning, itching Heavy yellowish discharge	Bed rest and consultation with a Doctor.
Tumour or Sore in uterus	Lesions in uterus, Pain	Infection	A vaginal douche with water in which leaves of Neem boiled. Fomentation of lower abdomen and the pubes by cloth pad.
Dysmenorrhoea	Weakness and pain in groin proceeding menses	irritation in ovaries	Malfunctioning of ovaries
Metritis	Inflammation of uterus	Intenral Inflammation	-do-
Sterlity	unable to conceive	Malfunctioning of reproductive organs	Have treatment of Anaemia and nutriteous diet.

Index

B

C

R

S

T

U

V

W

Y